Wide Angle Health

This EMF resource document began with the intent to answer the 110 left⸍ ⸍⸍⸍⸍⸍⸍ questions from the audience at the Commonwealth Club's panel, **"Microwave Radiation: The Shadow Side of the Wireless Revolution"**, which we did not get a chance to answer that evening. It has expanded organically beyond that to offer citizens everywhere a broad understanding of the importance of electromagnetic factors in health, a candid discussion of the failings of our government leading to this very serious man-made public health issue and our best recommendations for how to protect your family's health in high EMF environments, at least until biologically-based exposure standards are established.

Many thanks to the Commonwealth Club for hosting this panel on microwave radiation, and to Edward F. Adams who, on founding the Commonwealth Club in 1903, declared "We only propose to find truth and turn it loose in the world." Those words have inspired us.

Gratitude to co-panelists David Carpenter, MD and Cindy Sage, MA, Co-Editors of the landmark BioInitiative Report, for exceptional presentations on the panel that evening, and to Prof. Magda Havas, PhD, who tirelessly labored with me to produce this post-event Q&A document, **"Public Health SOS: The Shadow Side of the Wireless Revolution"**. We hope the education contained herein will serve as a tremendous value to citizens at a time when there is a vacuum in the marketplace for information on this important public health topic.

Special thanks go to William Grant, PhD, Chair of the Commonwealth Club's Health & Medicine Forum, and Kerry Curtis, Chair of its Environment & Natural Resources Forum, for understanding the importance of this topic and seeing that the program get on the calendar at our country's premier public affairs venue. Also thanks to Chantel Benson, Riki Rafner and all other Commonwealth Club staff who made this event a huge success, and to those who later made sure the audio recording of the program was included in the Commonwealth Club's permanent podcast archive and aired in entirety on public radio in San Francisco. We appreciate the staff's commitment to the Club's original mission.

Finally, many thanks go to the dedicated scientists who reviewed this document, sometimes several times, and always in the same selfless spirit of community service with which we are creating this document for you. And, to the many other experts we consulted, many of whom have been in this field for decades, who readily took the time to contribute to various sections when asked. This could not have been done without you!

Please forgive us if any of our answers seem incomplete, or if you wanted further detail. We have done our best given time constraints and natural limits on our knowledge! We hope **"Public Health SOS: The Shadow Side of the Wireless Revolution"** gives readers enough information to become their own best environmental detective, health preservation guide and advocate for electromagnetic health in communities across America. And, that it inspires journalists everywhere to look at the facts on this issue—and to pursue the hundreds of story themes herein!

Camilla Rees

Camilla Rees
CEO, Wide Angle Health, LLC

Radiofrequency Towers and Antennas Across the U.S.

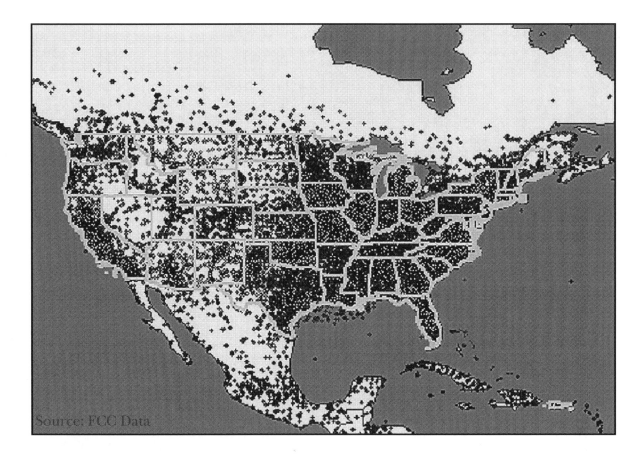

Source: FCC Data

The proliferation of electromagnetic fields in America is known by scientists to be significantly compromising the health of humans, animals and nature.

It is time for us as a society to acknowledge the health consequences of radiation emitting telecommunications technologies, electronic equipment, energy efficient lighting and radiofrequency-based technologies increasingly used by electric utilities, and to take steps to protect health.

Physicians, parents, schools, employers, real estate professionals and government officials at every level must become educated on this important emerging public health issue.

This is an educational document about an important public health issue. It is not to be construed as medical advice. For individual health issues or concerns, please see your physician or other licensed health practitioner.

"Public Health SOS: The Shadow Side of the Wireless Revolution"

A Resource for Concerned Citizens

Section I: Are You Sensitive to Electromagnetic Energy?

We begin with a checklist summarizing exactly what is happening to peoples' health globally from exposure to electromagnetic fields. This is a useful section to catch potential symptoms early so you can take steps to remediate your environment.

Section II: Expressions of Concern from Scientists, Physicians, Health Policy Experts & Others

Hear concerns about electromagnetic pollution from experts. The public's support is called for now so our government pays attention to this important public health issue and changes currently non-protective exposure guidelines to be protective of humans, animals, and nature.

Section III: Electromagnetic (EMF) Safety Recommendations

The bottom line on EMF safety—learn what's important for your family, community and employer to know in order to protect your health as well as possible.

Section IV: "110 Questions on Electromagnetic Pollution"

Commentary on typical EMF-related questions in the minds of the public and the media raised by the audience at the Commonwealth Club of California. Includes links to research and references. Rationale behind the 'Electromagnetic Safety Recommendations' described in Section III are discussed in more detail.

Section V: Books, Videos, Journals and Websites, Etc.

Points you to exactly where you need to go to learn more about electromagnetic factors in health.

Section VI: Community Health Survey

Consider conducting the *Green Audit* health survey in your community before, and then after, Wi-Max or Broadband Over Power lines rolls out, or before a tower goes up in your neighborhood. Services of an epidemiologist advised.

Section VII: Links to Petitions

1) **Petition to Congress** (www.ElectromagneticHealth.org)
2) **The BioInitiative Report** (www.bioinitiative.org)
3) **The Venice Resolution** (www.icems.eu)

Section VIII: How to Support Further EMF Advocacy & Research

Wide Angle Health

"...All communication in the body eventually takes place via very subtle electromagnetic signaling between cells that is now being disrupted by artificial electropollution we have not had time to adapt to. As Alvin Toffler emphasized in Future Shock, too much change in too short a time produces severe stress due to adaptational failure. The adverse effects of electrosmog may take decades to be appreciated, although some, like carcinogenicity, are already starting to surface. This gigantic experiment on our children and grandchildren could result in massive damage to mind and body with the potential to produce a disaster of unprecedented proportions, unless proper precautions are immediately implemented."

— Paul J. Rosch, MD
Clinical Professor of Medicine and Psychiatry, New York Medical College; Diplomat, National Board of Medical Examiners

Section I: Are You Sensitive to Electromagnetic Energy?
- By Dr. Magda Havas, PhD

Those who suffer from electrohypersensitivity (EHS) have the following reactions to . . .

1. **EMFs in stores (due to wireless communications, security systems and lighting)**
   - confusion and poor short-term memory, also called "brain fog," so they go shopping with list in hand and spend as little time in the store as possible. Some can't recall where they parked their car.
   - headache that becomes progressively worse the more time they spend in the store
   - dizziness, numbness, tremors, and other neurological disorders
   - nausea or feeling unwell
   - fatigue and weakness
   - problems with vision and hearing (buzzing in ears)
   - depression, anxiety, and other mood disorders

2. **Mobile phones (both cell phones and cordless phones)**
   - feeling of warmth
   - numbness in fingers
   - facial flushing on the side of the head where the phone is held
   - headaches that become progressively worse and last longer with continued phone use
   - eventually some cannot be in the same room when others are talking on a cell phone
   - dizziness, nausea, chest pain, shortness of breath
   - deafness, blurred vision, blistering skin and strokes have all been reported
   - severely affected people can not use a cell phone at all (extreme pain, loss of muscular control)

3. **Some energy efficient light bulbs, especially compact fluorescent lights (CFL)**
   - headaches and other body aches
   - confusion and memory loss, "brain fog"
   - fatigue
   - dizziness, nausea, feeling unwell
   - eye problems including eye strain leading to dry eyes or watery eyes, problems with vision, tired eyes
   - ringing in the ears (similar to tinnitus)
   - skin problems including any combination of rashes, itchiness, blotchiness
   - depression, anxiety, and other mood disorders
   - arthritic pains

If you checked several categories above, you may be electro-magnetically sensitive.

Most people associate symptoms like these with aging or living a stressful life-style, which may be the case, but for EHS sufferers, if they pay attention, they often find that their symptoms become worse in environments with higher EMF exposure. As time goes on, they may find that they respond faster to electromagnetic exposures, that their reactions become more severe, and that it takes them longer to recover (return to "normal").

Symptoms of Electrohypersensitivity or Radio Wave Sickness

Neurological: headaches, dizziness, nausea, difficulty concentrating, memory loss, irritability, depression, anxiety, insomnia, fatigue, weakness, tremors, muscle spasms, numbness, tingling, altered reflexes, muscle and joint paint, leg/foot pain, flu-like symptoms, fever. More severe reactions can include seizures, paralysis, psychosis and stroke.

Cardiac: palpitations, arrhythmias, pain or pressure in the chest, low or high blood pressure, slow or fast heart rate, shortness of breath

Respiratory: sinusitis, bronchitis, pneumonia, and asthma

Dermatological: skin rash, itching, burning, and facial flushing

Ophthalmologic: pain or burning in the eyes, pressure in/behind the eyes, deteriorating vision, floaters, and cataracts

Others: digestive problems; abdominal pain; enlarged thyroid, testicular/ovarian pain; dryness of lips, tongue, mouth, eyes; great thirst; dehydration; nosebleeds; internal bleeding; altered sugar metabolism; immune abnormalities; redistribution of metals within the body; hair loss; pain in the teeth; deteriorating fillings; impaired sense of smell; ringing in the ears.

Between 3% and 35% of the population may have symptoms of EHS according to The Power Watch Handbook by Alasdair and Jean Philips.

Common Sources of Radio Waves (wired & wireless)

Outdoors: broadcast and cell phone antennas, radar, cell phones, pagers systems, two-way radios, Wi-Fi antennas.

Indoors: cordless telephones and their base units, wireless computers and their wireless routers, wired computers, televisions, microwave ovens, dimmer switches, security systems, fax machines, answering machines, assistive listening systems and devices for the hearing impaired, wireless microphones, variable speed motors, transformers, wireless child monitors, electric utility smart meters, signal-broadcasting smoke alarms, some electronic games . . .

Vehicles: CB radios, ignition systems, spark plugs, alternators, mobile radar units; electric trains and subways.

Section II: Expressions of Concern from Scientists, Physicians, Health Policy Experts & Others

William Rea, MD
Founder & Director of the Environmental Health Center, Dallas
Past President, American Academy of Environmental Medicine

"Sensitivity to electromagnetic radiation is the emerging health problem of the 21st century. It is imperative health practitioners, governments, schools and parents learn more about it. The human health stakes are significant."

Olle Johansson, Ph.D.
Associate Professor, The Experimental Dermatology Unit, Department of Neuroscience, Karolinska Institute, Stockholm, Sweden

"It is evident that various biological alterations, including immune system modulation, are present in electrohypersensitive persons. There must be an end to the pervasive nonchalance, indifference and lack of heartfelt respect for the plight of these persons. It is clear something serious has happened and is happening. Every aspect of electrohypersensitive peoples' lives, including the ability to work productively in society, have healthy relations and find safe, permanent housing, is at stake. The basics of life are becoming increasingly inaccessible to a growing percentage of the world's population. I strongly advise all governments to take the issue of electromagnetic health hazards seriously and to take action while there is still time. There is too great a risk that the ever increasing RF-based communications technologies represent a real danger to humans, especially because of their exponential, ongoing and unchecked growth. Governments should act decisively to protect public health by changing the exposure standards to be biologically-based, communicating the results of the independent science on this topic and aggressively researching links with a multitude of associated medical conditions."

Magda Havas, PhD
Associate Professor, Environment & Resource Studies, Trent University, Canada.
Expert in radiofrequency radiation, electromagnetic fields, dirty electricity and ground current.

"Radio frequency radiation and other forms of electromagnetic pollution are harmful at orders of magnitude well below existing guidelines. Science is one of the tools society uses to decide health policy. In the case of telecommunications equipment, such as cell phones, wireless networks, cell phone antennas, PDAs, and portable phones, the science is being ignored. Current guidelines urgently need to be re-examined by government and reduced to reflect the state of the science. There is an emerging public health crisis at hand and time is of the essence."

David Carpenter, MD

Professor, Environmental Health Sciences, and Director, Institute for Health and the Environment, School of Public Health, University of Albany, SUNY
Co-Editor, The BioInitiative Report (www.BioInitiative.org)

"Electromagnetic fields are packets of energy that does not have any mass, and visible light is what we know best. X-rays are also electromagnetic fields, but they are more energetic than visible light. Our concern is for those electromagnetic fields that are less energetic than visible light, including those that are associated with electricity and those used for communications and in microwave ovens. The fields associated with electricity are commonly called "extremely low frequency" fields (ELF), while those used in communication and microwave ovens are called "radiofrequency" (RF) fields. Studies of people have shown that both ELF and RF exposures result in an increased risk of cancer, and that this occurs at intensities that are too low to cause tissue heating. Unfortunately, all of our exposure standards are based on the false assumption that there are no hazardous effects at intensities that do not cause tissue heating. Based on the existing science, many public health experts believe it is possible we will face an epidemic of cancers in the future resulting from uncontrolled use of cell phones and increased population exposure to Wi-Fi and other wireless devices. Thus it is important that all of us, and especially children, restrict our use of cell phones, limit exposure to background levels of Wi-Fi, and that government and industry discover ways in which to allow use of wireless devices without such elevated risk of serious disease. We need to educate decision-makers that 'business as usual' is unacceptable. The importance of this public health issue can not be underestimated."

Martin Blank, PhD

Associate Professor, Department of Physiology and Cellular BioPhysics,
Columbia University, College of Physicians and Surgeons; Researcher in Bioelectromagnetics;
Author of the BioInitiative Report's section on Stress Proteins.

"Cells in the body react to EMFs as potentially harmful, just like to other environmental toxins, including heavy metals and toxic chemicals. The DNA in living cells recognizes electromagnetic fields at very low levels of exposure; and produces a biochemical stress response. The scientific evidence tells us that our safety standards are inadequate, and that we must protect ourselves from exposure to EMF due to power lines, cell phones and the like, or risk the known consequences. The science is very strong and we should sit up and pay attention."

Whitney North Seymour, Jr., Esq.
Co-Founder Natural Resources Defense Council;
Retired Attorney; Former New York State Senator & United States Attorney,
Southern District of NY

"Electromagnetic radiation is a very serious human and environmental health issue that needs immediate attention by Congress. The BioInitiative Report is a major milestone in understanding the health risks from wireless technology. Every responsible elected official owes it to his or her constituents to learn and act on its finding and policy recommendations."

B. Blake Levitt
Former *New York Times* writer and author of "*Electromagnetic Fields, A Consumer's Guide to the Issues and How to Protect Ourselves*", and Editor of "*Cell Towers, Wireless Convenience? Or Environmental Hazard?*"

"Ambient man-made electromagnetic fields (EMFs), across a range of frequencies, are a serious environmental issue. Yet most environmentalists know little about it, perhaps because the subject has been the purview of physicists and engineers for so long that biologists have lost touch with electromagnetism's fundamental inclusion in the biological paradigm. All living cells and indeed whole living beings, no matter what genus or species, are dynamic coherent electrical systems utterly reliant on bioelectricity for life's most basic metabolic processes. It turns out that most living things are fantastically sensitive to vanishingly small EMF exposures. Living cells interpret such exposures as part of our normal cellular activities (think heartbeats, brainwaves, cell division itself, etc.) The problem is, man-made electromagnetic exposures aren't "normal." They are artificial artifacts, with unusual intensities, signaling characteristics, pulsing patterns, and wave forms, that don't exist in nature. And they can misdirect cells in myriad ways. Every aspect of the ecosystem may be affected, including all living species from animals, humans, plants and even microorganisms in water and soil. We are already seeing problems in sentinel species like birds, bats, and bees. Wildlife is known to abandon areas when cell towers are placed. Radiofrequency radiation (RF)—the part of the electromagnetic spectrum used in all-things-wireless today—is a known immune system suppressor, among other things. RF is a form of energetic air pollution and we need to understand it as such. Humans are not the only species being affected. The health of our planet may be in jeopardy from this newest environmental concern—added to all the others. Citizens need to call upon government to fund appropriate research and to get industry influence out of the dialogue. We ignore this at our own peril now."

Eric Braverman, MD

Brain researcher, author of *The Edge Effect* and Director of Path Medical in New York City and The PATH Foundation. Expert in the brain's global impact on illness and health.

"There is no question EMFs have a major effect on neurological functioning. They slow our brain waves and affect our long-term mental clarity. We should minimize exposures as much as possible to optimize neurotransmitter levels and prevent deterioration of health."

Abraham R. Liboff, PhD

Research Professor, Center for Molecular Biology and Biotechnology
Florida Atlantic University, Boca Raton, Florida
Co-Editor, *Electromagnetic Biology and Medicine*

"The key point about electromagnetic pollution that the public has to realize is that it is not necessary that the intensity be large for a biological interaction to occur. There is now considerable evidence that extremely weak signals can have physiological consequences. These interactive intensities are about 1000 times smaller than the threshold values formerly estimated by otherwise knowledgeable theoreticians, who, in their vainglorious approach to science, rejected all evidence to the contrary as inconsistent with their magnificent calculations. These faulty estimated thresholds are yet to be corrected by both regulators and the media.

The overall problem with environmental electromagnetism is much deeper, not only of concern at power line frequencies, but also in the radiofrequency range encompassing mobile phones. Here the public's continuing exposure to electromagnetic radiation is largely connected to money. Indeed the tens of billions of dollars in sales one finds in the cell phone industry makes it mandatory to corporate leaders that they deny, in knee-jerk fashion, any indication of hazard.

There may be hope for the future in knowing that weakly intense electromagnetic interactions can be used for good as well as harm. The fact that such fields are biologically effective also implies the likelihood of medical applications, something that is now taking place. As this happens, I think it will make us more aware about how our bodies react to electromagnetism, and it should become even clearer to everyone concerned that there is reason to be very, very careful about ambient electromagnetic fields."

Lennart Hardell, MD, PhD

Professor at University Hospital, Orebro, Sweden.
World-renowned expert on cell phones, cordless phones, brain tumors, and the safety
of wireless radiofrequency and microwave radiation.
Member, BioInitiative Working Group

"The evidence for risks from prolonged cell phone and cordless phone use is quite
strong when you look at people who have used these devices for 10 years or
longer, and when they are used mainly on one side of the head. Recent studies
that do not report increased risk of brain tumors and acoustic neuromas have not
looked at heavy users, use over ten years or longer, and do not look at the part of
the brain which would reasonably have exposure to produce a tumor."

Samuel Milham MD, MPH

Medical epidemiologist in occupational epidemiology.
First scientist to report increased leukemia and other cancers in electrical workers and to
demonstrate that the childhood age peak in leukemia emerged in conjunction with the spread
of residential electrification.

"Very recently, new research is suggesting that nearly all the human plagues
which emerged in the twentieth century, like common acute lymphoblastic
leukemia in children, female breast cancer, malignant melanoma and asthma,
can be tied to some facet of our use of electricity. There is an urgent need for
governments and individuals to take steps to minimize community and personal
EMF exposures."

Libby Kelley, MA

Managing Secretariat, International Commission For Electromagnetic Safety; Founder,
Council on Wireless Technology Impacts; Co-Producer of documentary, "*Public Exposure:
DNA, Democracy and the Wireless Revolution*"; EMF environmental consultant and leading
appellant in challenging the FCC Radio Frequency Radiation human exposure guidelines,
1997-2000.

"Radiofrequency radiation human exposure standards for personal wireless
communications devices and for environmental exposure to wireless
transmitters are set by national governments to guide the use of wireless
communications devices and for wireless transmitters. In the U.S., the Food and
Drug Administration and the Federal Communications Commission set these
standards. The International Commission For Electromagnetic Safety considers
these exposure standards to be inadequate as they are based on heating effects
and do not accommodate the low level, cumulative exposure conditions in which
the public now lives. These standards are also designed for acute, short term

exposure conditions and do not acknowledge the medical evidence pointing to increased risks and actual harm that results from chronic, intermittent exposure. Federal and State public health agencies are not officially addressing what many concerned scientists and medical doctors now see as an emerging public health problem. There are no health surveillance or remedial response systems in place to advise citizens about electromagnetic radiation exposure (EMR). As wireless technology evolves, ambient background levels increase, creating electrical pollution conditions which are becoming ubiquitous and more invasive. We strongly encourage consumers, manufacturers, utility providers and policymakers to reduce, eliminate and mitigate EMR exposure conditions and to support biologically based standards."

James S. Turner, Esq.
Chairman of the Board, Citizens for Health
Partner, Swankin & Turner, Washington, DC
Co-Author, "*Voice of the People: The Transpartisan Imperative in American Life*"

"According to the BioInitiative Report: A Rationale for a Biologically-Based Public Exposure Standard for Electromagnetic Fields—from electrical and electronic appliances, power lines and wireless devices such as cell phones, cordless phones, cellular antennas, towers, and broadcast transmission towers—we live in an invisible fog of EMF which thirty years of science, including over 2,000 peer reviewed studies, shows exposes us to serious health risks such as increased Alzheimer's disease, breast cancer, Lou Gehrig disease, EMF immune system hypersensitivity and disruption of brain function and DNA. The public needs to wake up politicians and public officials to the need for updating the decades old EMF public health standards. This report tells how."

Camilla Rees, MBA
CEO, Wide Angle Health, LLC
Patient education and advocacy

"The U.S. spends over $2 trillion dollars on health care each year, of which about 78% is from people with chronic illnesses, without adequately exploring and understanding what factors—including EMF/RF—contribute to imbalances in peoples' bodies' in the first place. After reading The BioInitiative Report on the biological effects of electromagnetic radiation, it should come as no surprise to policymakers, given continually increasing levels of EMF/RF exposures in our environment, that close to 50% of Americans now live with a chronic illness. This percentage will certainly increase with increasing levels of electrosmog from cell phones, Wi-Fi, Wi-Max, Broadband Over Power lines, uncontained ground current, etc. It is imperative our government leaders become more cognizant of the role electromagnetic factors are playing in the incidence of disease, health care costs, and in the erosion of quality of life and productivity in America."

L. Lloyd Morgan, BS Electronic Engineering

Director, Central Brain Tumor Registry of the United States;
Member, Bioelectromagnetics Society; Member Brain Tumor Epidemiological Consortium*

"There is every indication that cell phones cause brain tumors, salivary gland tumors and eye cancer. Yet, because the cell phone industry provides a substantial proportion of research funding, this reality is hidden from the general public. The Interphone Study, a 13-country research project, substantially funded by the cell phone industry, has consistently shown that use of a cell phone protects the user from risk of a brain tumor! Does anything more need to be said? It is time that fully independent studies be funded by those governmental agencies whose charter is to protect its citizens so that the truth about the very damaging health hazards of microwave radiation becomes clear and well known."

Janet Newton

President, The EMR Policy Institute
www.EMRPolicy.org

"The radiofrequency radiation safety policy in force in the United States fails to protect the public. Currently in the US there are more than 260 million wireless subscribers, the demand that drives the continuing build-out of antenna sites in residential and commercial neighborhoods, including near schools, daycare centers, and senior living centers and in the workplace. The January 2008 report issued by the National Academy of Sciences committee whose task was to examine the needs and gaps in the research on the biological effects of exposure to these antennas points out that the research studies to date do not adequately represent exposure realities. Specifically, the studies 1) assume a single antenna rather than the typical arrangements of a minimum of four to six antennas per site, thereby underestimating exposure intensities, 2) do not pertain to the commonly used multiple-element base station antennas, thereby not taking into account exposures to multiple frequencies, 3) lack models of several heights for men, women, and children of various ages for use in the characterization of Specific Absorption Rate (SAR) distributions for exposures from cell phones, wireless PCs, and base stations and 4) do not take into consideration absorption effects of exposures from the many different radio frequency emitting devices to which the public is often simultaneously exposed. A federal research strategy to address these very serious inadequacies in the science on which our government is basing health policy is sorely needed now."

---

* For identification purposes only: All statements are mine and mine alone and do not represent positions or opinions of the Central Brain Tumor Registry of the United States, the Bioelectromagnetics Society or the Brain Tumor Epidemiological Consortia

Professor Livio Giuliani, PhD

Spokesperson, International Commission for Electromagnetic Safety (www.icems.eu);
Deputy Director, Italian National Institute for Worker Protection and Safety, East Venice and
South Tyrol; Professor, School of Biochemistry of Camerino University, Italy

"The Venice Resolution, initiated by the International Commission for
Electromagnetic Safety (ICEMS) on June 6, 2008, and signed by peer reviewed
scientists worldwide, states in part, "We are compelled to confirm the existence
of non-thermal effects of electromagnetic fields on living matter, which seem to
occur at every level of investigation from molecular to epidemiological. Recent
epidemiological evidence is stronger than before. We recognize the growing
public health problem known as electrohypersensitivity. We strongly advise
limited use of cell phones, and other similar devices, by young children and
teenagers, and we call upon governments to apply the Precautionary Principle
as an interim measure while more biologically relevant exposure standards are
developed."

Paul J. Rosch, MD

Clinical Professor of Medicine and Psychiatry, New York Medical College;
Honorary Vice President, International Stress Management Association; Diplomate, National
Board of Medical Examiners; Full Member, Russian Academy of Medical Sciences; Fellow, The
Royal Society of Medicine; Emeritus Member, The Bioelectromagnetics Society

"Claims that cell phones pose no health hazards are supported solely by Specific
Absorption Rate (SAR) limits safety standards written by the telecommunications
industry decades ago based on studies they funded. These have made the
erroneous assumption that the only harm that could come from cell phone
radiofrequency emissions would be from a thermal or heating action, since
such non thermal fields can have no biological effects. The late Dr. Ross
Adey disproved this three decades ago by demonstrating that very similar
radiofrequency fields with certain carrier and modulation frequencies that had
insufficient energy to produce any heating could cause the release of calcium
ions from cells. Since then, numerous research reports have confirmed that non
thermal fields from cell phones, tower transmitters, power lines, and other man
made sources can significantly affect various tissues and physiologic functions.
We are constantly being bathed in an increasing sea of radiation from exposure
to the above, as well as electrical appliances, computers, Bluetooth devices,
Wi-Fi installations and over 2,000 communications satellites in outer space that
shower us with signals to GPS receivers.

New Wi-Max transmitters on cell phone towers that have a range of up to two
square miles compared to Wi-Fi's 300 feet will soon turn the core of North
America into one huge electromagnetic hot spot. Children are more severely
affected because their brains are developing and their skulls are thinner.
A two-minute call can alter brain function in a child for an hour, which is why

other countries ban their sale or discourage their use under the age of 18. In contrast, this is the segment of the population now being targeted here in a $2 billion U.S. advertising campaign that views "tweens" (children between 8 and 12 years old) as the next big cell phone market. Firefly and Barbie cell phones are also being promoted for 6 to 8-year-olds.

It is not generally appreciated that there is a cumulative effect and that talking on a cell phone for just an hour a day for ten years can add up to 10,000 watts of radiation. That's ten times more than from putting your head in a microwave oven. Pregnant women may also be at increased risk based on a study showing that children born to mothers who used a cell phone just two or three times a day during pregnancy showed a dramatic increase in hyperactivity and other behavioral and emotional problems. And for the 30% of children who had also used a cell phone by age 7, the incidence of behavioral problems was 80% higher! Whether ontogeny (embryonic development) recapitulates phylogeny is debatable, but it is clear that lower forms of life are also much more sensitive. If you put the positive electrode of a 1.5 volt battery in the Pacific Ocean at San Francisco and the negative one off San Diego, sharks in between these cities can detect the few billionths of a volt electrical field. EMF fields have also been implicated in the recent massive but mysterious disappearance of honeybee colonies essential for pollinating over 90 commercial crops. As Albert Einstein warned, "If the bee disappeared off the surface of the globe, then man would only have four years of life left."

Finally, all life on earth evolved under the influence of solar radiation and geomagnetic forces that we have learned to adapt to and in some instances even utilize. The health of all living systems (ranging upward from a cell, tissue, organ or person, to a family, organization or nation) depends on good communication – good communication within, as well as with the external environment. All communication in the body eventually takes place via very subtle electromagnetic signaling between cells that is now being disrupted by artificial electropollution we have not had time to adapt to. As Alvin Toffler emphasized in Future Shock, too much change in too short a time produces severe stress due to adaptational failure. The adverse effects of electrosmog may take decades to be appreciated, although some, like carcinogenicity, are already starting to surface. This gigantic experiment on our children and grandchildren could result in massive damage to mind and body with the potential to produce a disaster of unprecedented proportions, unless proper precautions are immediately implemented. At the same time, we must acknowledge that novel electromagnetic therapies have been shown to benefit stress related disorders ranging from anxiety, depression and insomnia, to arthritis, migraine and tension headaches. As demonstrated in Bioelectromagnetic Medicine, they may also be much safer and more effective than drugs, so we need to avoid throwing the baby out with the bathwater."

Professor Jacqueline McGlade

Executive Director, European Environmental Agency
Advisor to European Union countries under the European Commission

"There are many examples of the failure to use the precautionary principle in the past, which have resulted in serious and often irreversible damage to health and environments. Appropriate, precautionary and proportionate actions taken now to avoid plausible and potentially serious threats to health from EMF are likely to be seen as prudent and wise from future perspectives."

European Parliament, September 2008

"The limits on exposure to electromagnetic fields which have been set for the general public are obsolete."

After reading these quotes, please consider signing ElectromagneticHealth.org's Petition to Congress at www.ElectromagneticHealth.org.

The Petition asks Congress to:

1. **Mandate the Federal Communications Commission (FCC) revisit its exposure guidelines for radiofrequency radiation (RF) immediately.**

2. **Repeal Section 704 of the Telecommunications Act of 1996, which took away the rights of state and local governments to stop the erection of cell towers and wireless antennas in their communities based on "environmental" grounds (defined by FCC as "human health").**

3. **Declare a national moratorium on further wireless infrastructure build-out, including the Wi-Max roll-out currently underway.**

4. **Establish cell phone and wireless-free neighborhoods, transportation options, government buildings, and public spaces; require employers to establish wireless free zones; and, mandate the removal of cellular and wireless technologies from public schools and their properties.**

Please sign the petition at www.ElectromagneticHealth.org

Technological Advances
Extremely Low Frequency (ELF) to Radio Frequency (RF)

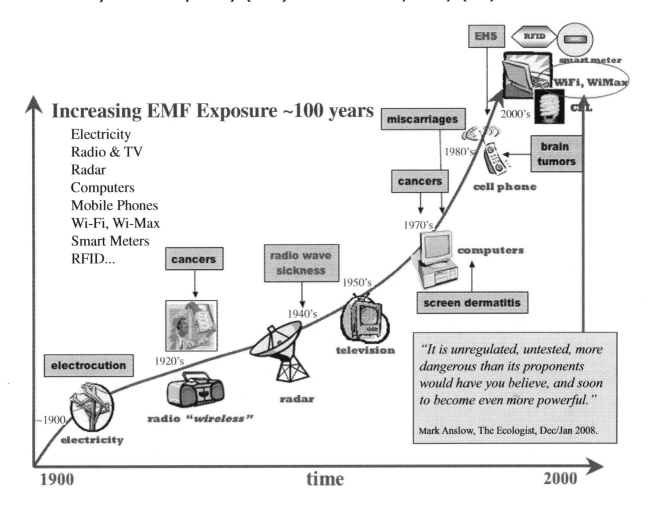

Increasing EMF Exposure ~100 years

Electricity
Radio & TV
Radar
Computers
Mobile Phones
Wi-Fi, Wi-Max
Smart Meters
RFID...

EHS RFID smart meter

WiFi, WiMax

2000's CFL

miscarriages

1980's

brain tumors

cancers cell phone

1970's computers

radio wave sickness

1950's screen dermatitis

cancers

1940's

1920's television

electrocution

radar

"It is unregulated, untested, more dangerous than its proponents would have you believe, and soon to become even more powerful."

Mark Anslow, The Ecologist, Dec/Jan 2008.

~1900 radio *"wireless"*

electricity

1900   time   2000

Extremely-Low Frequency (ELF) and Radiofrequency (RF) Electromagnetic Fields Have Very Similar Biological Effects

- Genetic Effects
- Cancer
- Cellular/Molecular Effects
- Electrophysiology
- Behavior
- Nervous System
- Blood-brain barrier
- Calcium
- Cardiovascular
- Warm sensation
- Hormones
- Immunology
- Metabolic rate/effects
- Reproduction/growth
- Subjective symptoms
- Stress

Source: Dr. Henry Lai, Research Professor, Department of Bioengineering, University of Washington. Presentation March 21, 2008 at Council on Wireless Technology Impacts EMF Panel, San Francisco, CA.

Section III: Electromagnetic Safety Recommendations

These safety suggestions are based on a large and growing body of research showing a potential connection between EMF and many health challenges. Key research is referenced throughout the next section, Section IV, "110 Questions on Electromagnetic Pollution." This, Section III, is a summary section intended to give you the bottom line on how you might change your lifestyle to reflect both common sense and what the science shows.

Cell Phone/Cordless Phones

Do not use a cell phone unless is it essential and then speak for as short a time as possible. View your cell phone as something for emergencies only. Use the speaker phone whenever possible to keep the phone away from your skull and your body. If this is not possible, use a pneumatic (plastic air-tube) earpiece to reduce the radiation to your brain. Never keep a cell phone or PDA unit against your body when turned on, and do not spend unnecessary time playing games, sending text messages or connecting to the internet in this way.

Wean yourself off your cell phone. When you find you are able to do your business without one, consider giving it up completely unless you feel you need it for emergencies.

Same goes for cordless phones—most emit radiofrequency radiation 24/7. Replace them with landline phones. Get a long cord if it's necessary for you to walk around your house while talking on the phone. If you must use a cordless phone, just as with cell phones, limit the number of calls and the duration and use the pneumatic (plastic air tube) earpiece. Ensure your cordless phone is not a "DECT" phone (Digitally Enhanced Communications Technology) which radiates you and your home or office 24/7 whether you are using the phone or not.

Wired *or* wireless headsets with cell phones are not considered adequate protection. According to a University of York study wired headsets reduce radiation at the head significantly, but note the wire in a wired headset will still transmit the radiation along your body like an antenna, and the phone still emits radiation in your hand and/or near other body parts, such as your stomach, abdomen, kidneys, reproductive organs, etc. And, wireless headsets bring the addition of wireless frequencies right into, or onto, your ear. In both instances, your body is still being exposed to the cell phone radiation from the phone, just not at the level of the head. It's best to use the speakerphone, placed very far away from your body, or otherwise, to use the air tube headset with an additional extension cord to place the phone as far away from your body as possible.

At times when your full attention is important, and especially for long calls, always use a landline phone.

Do not allow children to use cell phones. According to the Chairman of the Russian National Committee on Non-Ionizing Radiation Protection 1) the absorption of electromagnetic energy is higher in a child's head, 2) they are more sensitive to this energy, 3) they are more sensitive to the accumulation of adverse effects under conditions of chronic exposure, and 4) EMF affects the formation of the higher nervous system activity. The Committee recommends 'urgency' to protect children's health from the influence of EMF from mobile communication. Research reported at the 1st international conference on mobile phones and health held at the Royal Society in London in September 2008 indicates that children and teenagers are five times more likely to get brain cancer if they use mobile phones. This risk may be underestimated because the study does not show the risks of phone use over many years. And the risk to young people using cordless phones was almost as great, at four times higher risk of brain cancer.

Pregnant women or those trying to conceive should minimize use of a cell phone, and not be around other people using them. Special attention to EMF safety of the sleeping location of pregnant women is also advised. A recent pilot research study has shown higher rates of babies born with autism where the mothers' sleeping locations had high levels of RF electromagnetic radiation. Also, in a very large, research study of 13,000 children at UCLA and Aarhus, Denmark, it has been shown that when women use mobile phones when pregnant just two or three times a day, the risk of their babies developing hyperactivity and difficulties with conduct, emotions and relationships by the time they reach school age increases over 50%, and when those children also later used the phones they were 80% more likely to suffer from difficulties with behavior (*Epidemiology*, July 2008).

Always turn off your cell phone at night. Never leave the phone anywhere near your head at night, if it needs to be kept on in an emergency.

If you use a mobile phone in public be respectful of other people as radiation from your phone is impacting others, too. Some people are especially sensitive, and some severely affected. Step well away from others (15 feet or more) to place your call. Turn off your phone completely after the call, as if it is on standby it is still impacting others who may be near you. Also, do not leave your cell phone turned on in meetings where it could affect the ability of others to focus. And do not use your mobile phone regularly in an office environment where it could be impacting others in nearby offices. Be considerate—and realize you are a source of debilitating radiation for some people. The same courtesy should be extended for cordless phones. If you share a residence, replace cordless phones with landline phones.

Never use a cell phone while driving. Make sure to turn the phone completely off when in the car. Not only is one exposed to the brain altering effects of the frequencies, but to what is called "cognitive capture", when one's mind and emotions are preoccupied with the call and not the road. 45 countries today ban cell phone use while driving (http://www.cellularnews.com/car_bans/). Also, realize exposure levels are much higher while driving because of the ongoing cell reconnection as your vehicle moves forward, and because of the internal reflections in the metal vehicle. Pull over or into a parking lot to check your messages and return your calls. Insist any passengers not use a cell phone while you are driving, and inform children and other passengers of the dangers of cell phone use while driving. For similar reasons, do not use cell phones in trains and elevators.

If you need to use your phone in the car, to minimize radiation ideally arrange to have the antenna hooked up outside the car. Absolutely do not use the phone while the car is in motion. Realize also that radiation from the phone in a car even while stationary will be reflected around inside the metal car, so even while your car is stopped talking on the phone inside a car is not ideal. Roll down the window to use the phone, at the very least.

Realize other drivers on the road are increasingly impaired by the short- and long-term effects of microwave radiation whether they know it or not, so drive defensively. Symptoms of impairment, including slowed reflexes, have been compared to drunk driving. If someone is using a cell phone in a car, note they are also irradiating everybody who is driving nearby, and also putting you at risk due to lack of full attention.

Wireless Exposures

Minimize exposure to wireless environments. Choose hard-wired connections at all times at home, both for your internet connection and between computer and printer. If you currently are using a wireless router, replace the wireless router with a hard-wired router. Run wiring from the router to the destinations where you use your computer. And if your computer comes standard with Wi-Fi capability, make sure to disable it. Unfortunately many printers today are Wi-Fi enabled with no means to disable it. Seek out printer brands where you know you can disable the Wi-Fi.

Minimize metal furniture, including mattresses with metal coils, as radiofrequency travels on (i.e. reflects from) metal and can create unknown hot spots. See "Passive Exposure to Mobile Phones: Enhancement of Intensity by Reflection." Go to http://www.beperkdestraling.org/Studies%20en%20Rapporten/Passive%20exposure%20mobile%20phones%20Journal%20Physical%20Society%20Japan%202007.pdf

Resist citywide Wi-Fi and/or Wi-Max. These create chronic 24/7 exposure for everyone. The health consequences of chronic wireless exposure can be significant, and severely debilitating for some people. Promote wired alternatives in your community such as fiber optic and hardwired cable, and educate your government officials on the important health differences. Refer them to the BioInitiative Report (www.BioInitiative.org) to read a review of over 2,000 research studies on EMF.

Wi-Max (or long distance Wi-Fi that spreads microwave radiation over many miles) must be stopped before it is rolled out across America in major metropolitan areas covering half of America in the next 2 years. Otherwise, one can expect an exodus from urban areas, as the estimated 3-8% of the population seriously impacted by this form of radiation will not be able to tolerate it, the 35% moderately impacted will become worse and want to move, and other informed parties will choose to migrate to remote areas, including to countries that are now lowering exposure guidelines, for prevention.

Choose hotels with hard-wired connections in the bedrooms or no internet at all to get well rested. Alternatively, find a green B&B or simple retreat center without wireless. You will sleep better in non-wireless environments. Travel with Graham-Stetzer filters to minimize your exposure to dirty electricity in hotels if you find filtering in this way makes a positive difference for you. Professional athletes concerned about optimizing athletic performance, as well as some electrically sensitive people and business executives, will travel with a metal mesh tent they put over the bed to block out electromagnetic radiation. If the only option is a hotel with Wi-Fi, ask for a room as far away from the Wi-Fi transmitting equipment as possible and minimize the time you spend in the room.

Avoid wireless "hot spots" as much as possible, such as wireless internet cafes, supermarkets, mega stores and fast food chains with wireless. Stressing your body while digesting is particularly ill advised. Avoid flying on airlines that install wireless (several, including American Airlines, are said to be planning pilot programs.)

Shield yourself from neighborhood wireless networks. Look into RF shielding fabrics for curtains and RF shielding film for the windows. Go to www.EMFSafetyStore.com. Once a room has been shielded, it's important that you or your guests not operate RF emitting equipment inside this environment (e.g. cell phones, computers, cordless phones, microwave ovens, wireless indoor/outdoor thermometers, baby monitors, etc.) as this would be dangerous. Ideally, get the help of an EMF measurement expert who can first assess what kind of frequencies are actually present, and from what directions they are coming, in order to remediate effectively and cost efficiently.

Reduce Electric Fields

Unplug electric devices near beds. Do not use electric blankets, bedpads or waterbed heaters.

Use battery-powered digital alarm clocks. LCD displays are better than LED (where there is a glow). In all cases, keep clocks at a distance of at least 3 feet from the bed.

Eliminate extension cords and power strips near the bed.

For maximum rest, turn off the fuse box to your bedroom at night. You may be amazed at how much of a difference this can make in how rested you feel the next day! A 'demand switch' can be installed to turn off fuses from your bedside for convenience. For suppliers of demand switches and instructions for your electrician, email Info@ElectromagneticHealth.org.

Minimize "Dirty Power"

Avoid compact fluorescent bulbs. These bulbs emit radiofrequency radiation, UV radiation and dirty electricity, otherwise known as high frequency transients. They also contain mercury, which is a serious health hazard if broken. Keep using incandescent bulbs. Or use LED bulbs instead, which in many instances are even more energy efficient than Compact Fluorescents, and preferably CLEDs which have no transformer converting from AC to DC. In conventional LEDs and CFLs, this process generates dirty electricity. CLEDs operate directly on AC current, using less power and no toxic chemicals.

Use Graham-Stetzer filters in your electric outlets to buffer the dirty electricity (high frequency transients). Assess if you feel there has been an improvement, or if you may need other forms of remediation.

Eliminate dimmer switches. Dimmer switches generate dirty electricity. It is best to replace them with 3-way switches that also can reduce light intensity and are electromagnetically clean.

Reduce Magnetic Fields

Use flat screen LCD TVs and computer monitors. Avoid plasma TVs as they generate dirty electricity.

Fix any wiring problems causing unequal current flow.

Unplug electronic appliances when not in use.

Use battery based digital alarm clocks.

EMF Home Testing To Consider

Microwave Radiation (cell phone antennas, broadcast antennas, radar, wireless networks, DECT and other portable phones, wireless speakers, wireless baby monitors, wireless mice and keyboards, Bluetooth devices, "Smart" power systems, wireless thermometers and doorbells, etc.)

Electric & Magnetic fields (from home appliances, indoor wiring & plumbing, and, in the outdoors, from power lines, substations and their underground cables, sometimes transformers, and stray currents on underground water lines)

Power Quality on indoor electrical wiring (from appliances within home and from neighbors)

Ground Current (especially high frequencies) coming into home on plumbing fixtures.

Summary

In summary, given that ownership of cell phones and other wireless devices support a commercial infrastructure of towers and antennas impacting societal health as a whole, including species related issues such as DNA damage and impaired fertility, we recommend you get a land line phone, wean yourself off wireless technologies and take a stand for the electromagnetic health of yourself and your community.

The Electromagnetic Spectrum

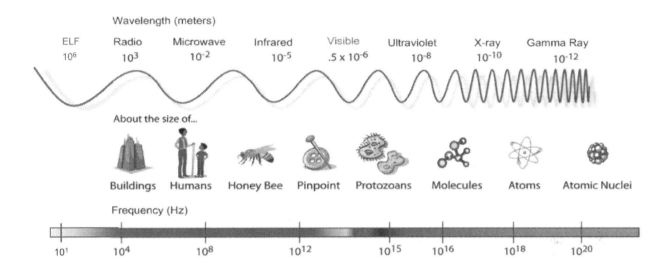

The electromagnetic spectrum above identifies the names given to the various regions of the spectrum along with their corresponding frequency (in cycles per second or Hertz) and wavelength (in meters).

The longest wavelengths and the slowest frequencies are referred to as **Extremely Low Frequency** or **ELF**. Electricity at 50/60 Hertz falls within this range as does brain wave activity (4-30 Hz) and heart rate (1- 2 Hz). The next band is called **Radio Frequency** and includes all forms of broadcast frequencies used for radio and television (thousands and millions Hz). **Microwave**, as the name implies, are smaller waves at higher frequencies (millions and billions Hz). Within this range we have mobile phones, microwave ovens, and radar. Above this region comes **infrared**, which we associated with heating. Some of our remote controls rely on infrared to turn TVs on and off and to change channels. **Visible light** is also part of the electromagnetic spectrum and it is the form of energy we are most familiar with because we can see it. **Ultraviolet radiation** is invisible to the human eye but can be "seen" by some species of insects. UV radiation can cause sunburn and damage DNA, which can lead to skin cancer, but also generates Vitamin D which has many very important health benefits. The radiation at and above **UV**, called **ionizing radiation**, is very dangerous. For that reason we limit human exposure to these frequencies and use them only when required for X-raying bone fractures or dental decay, for example.

Graphic source:
http://environmentaldefenseblogs.org/climate411/wpcontent/files/2007/07/ElectromagneticSpectrum.png, as modified by Dr. Havas

"... It turns out that most living things are fantastically sensitive to vanishingly small EMF exposures. Living cells interpret such exposures as part of our normal cellular activities (think heartbeats, brainwaves, cell division itself, etc.) The problem is, man-made electromagnetic exposures aren't "normal". They are artificial artifacts, with unusual intensities, signaling characteristics, pulsing patterns, and wave forms. And they can misdirect cells in myriad ways."

— B. Blake Levitt
Former *New York Times* writer and author of *"Electromagnetic Fields, A Consumer's Guide to the Issues and How to Protect Ourselves"*, and Editor of *"Cell Towers, Wireless Convenience? Or Environmental Hazard?"*

Section IV: 110 Questions from the Commonwealth Club's Panel "Microwave Radiation: The Shadow Side of the Wireless Revolution"*

Categories of Questions from the Audience

Random questions received from the Commonwealth Club audience have been grouped into loose categories. All questions we received from the audience are included here, thus you can expect some overlap.

- **Personal Safety**

- **Human Health**

- **Environmental Health**

- **Measuring Exposures & Exposure Standards**

- **Real Estate Related**

- **Science and Research Related**

- **Big Picture**

*To listen to the archived audio presentation "Microwave Radiation: The Shadow Side of the Wireless Revolution" given at The Commonwealth Club of California March 19, 2008, go to www.ElectromagneticHealth.org or purchase a CD from The Commonwealth Club at www.commonwealthclub.org.

"Throughout history, unintended consequences have frequently accompanied technological advances, such as with pharmaceutical, nuclear and coal mining technologies, for example, where there have been very serious human and environmental consequences, otherwise seen by society and scientists as 'advances'. Problems arise when there is a narrow focus on the technology, instead of appreciating the 'whole' impact. It is hard to put the brakes on once an industry is creating tremendous economic growth and jobs, and easier to put the blinders on, without very significant pressure from either consumers or government."

— Camilla Rees
Founder, ElectromagneticHealth.org
CEO, Wide Angle Health, LLC

110 Questions from the Commonwealth Club Audience

We highly recommend readers listen to the panel presentation from which the questions below were generated, found in the Commonwealth Club archives at http://www.commonwealthclub.org/archive/08/08-03microwaveradiation-audio.html or www.ElectromagneticHealth.org

Personal Safety

Cell & Portable Phone Use & Safety

#1. Is there a safe distance to hold a cell or portable phone away when using its speakerphone?

#2. Are the earpiece phones "safe"?

#3. My cordless phone is in my bedroom about 10' from my body when sleeping, is this distance safe?

#4. Do cell and portable phones affect us biologically if they are turned on but not being used?

#5. Regarding earpieces for cell phones, are wireless receivers even worse than putting the phone to your ear?

#6. What about Bluetooth headpieces—are they dangerous?

#7. Bluetooth headsets are radiating about 1 milligauss. Are they safe?

#8. Does it not stand to reason that Blue Tooth devices cause cancer as well? Is it not true that the wires in the headsets increase the danger not decrease it?

#9. How much effect does an ear phone have on the health effects of cell phones?

#10. What is more dangerous—the power or the frequencies of cell phones, or both?

Protection Devices—Do They Work?

#11. Do the small devices people attach to cell and cordless phones actually cut the EMF levels to a 'safe' limit?

#12. I have seen body pendants and whole house blockers of radiation. Are these legitimately helpful?

#13. Is there any product out there that we could use to protect us from EMR—for example, Teslar watches?

#14. Do you have any comment on WillauTronic products—esmog protection with transponder chip technology for cell phones, tvs, microwave ovens, cordless phones, etc? Or BioPro, Aegisguard, etc?

Home Health re. EMF/RF

#15. Are we more vulnerable while sleeping?

#16. Can you tell us about the risk and distance factors for having a Wi-Fi router or are you saying Wi-Fi is too dangerous to have in a house at all?

#17. What evidence is there for cumulative effects of microwave radiation from cell phones and Wi-Fi?

#18. Is there any risk standing near a microwave oven when it is operating? What distance?

#19. A friend uses a microwave with a cracked glass door, I told her not to, can you confirm the danger?

#20. What are the health effects of microwave ovens?

#21. Are energy efficient bulbs (i.e. Compact Fluorescent Bulbs) actually bad for our living space? Please elucidate.

#22. What is a safe level of EMF/RF to live with?

#23. Does having solar panels on a roof cause problems?

#24. Where do we get the filters to eliminate 'dirty electricity' on home and office wiring created by high RF environments? Are these considered legitimate as compared to the controversy around pendants that claim to be protective?

#25. Are TV remotes ELF transmitters?

#26. Can bed springs conduct these frequencies? What about metal furniture?

#27. What's the problem with plasma TVs?

#28. Where would we find the reflecting fabric? Does this protect from microwave radiation as well as from dirty electricity? Are there circumstances when it should not be used?

#29. Do you have any help to offer those of us fighting the installation of antenna towers (and labeled crazies)?

#30. How far away do cell phone towers have to be from your home to be 100% safe?

#31. What are you the panelists doing to reduce your own and your families' exposures to these hazards?

#32. Within months of installing a wireless internet network and wireless audio system in our house, mold developed. Is there any connection between wireless and mold?

#33. Do batteries emit less radiation than, say, electrical cords?

Automobiles

#34. Are cars equipped with Blue Tooth especially toxic?

#35. Are hybrid cars dangerous for our health? What levels of EMF exposure compared to non-hybrids?

Self-Protection While Traveling

#36. What should one do to combat the exposure in airplanes?

#37. What can I do to protect myself in a wireless hotel room so I don't awaken with brain fog? Are there any hotel chains that you know of not installing wireless in rooms?

#38. Some people feel worse around Wi-Fi. Is constant Wi-Fi exposure worse than cell phone radiation?

#39. Are there dangers in wearing clothing made of shielding fabrics? For example, if I wear a baseball cap made out of shielding material—I can understand it would shield my head from frequencies but what would happen to the frequencies that get into my body from elsewhere—do they get trapped in the brain area, becoming dangerous, because I am wearing the hat?

Human Health

Human Health Impacts of EMF/RF

#40. What are the common symptoms of microwave radiation exposure from cell phones, wireless etc?

#41. Dr. Olle Johansson has said that everyone exposed to EMFs registers an inflammatory reaction in the mast cells on the skin, whether or not they feel it. I think everyone is EMF sensitive and just vary in the disease of choice. Would this make sense?

#42. I find it terribly wrong the telecom industry has rights to affect my DNA. How much evidence is there that DNA is being impacted, and what are the known consequences of the DNA damage to date?

#43. How quickly does a cell phone affect the brain? Is it impacting its structure or function? Are the neurotransmitter levels affected—potentially linking wireless technologies to the depression epidemic?

#44. What are the consequences of the stated increased permeability of the blood-brain barrier?

#45. How much evidence is there linking EMF/RF to Parkinson's Disease?

#46. With autism now at epidemic levels—has a relationship between autism and ELF/EMF been studied?

#47. Do EMF exposures worsen reaction to toxic chemicals, mold and other allergens?

#48. Can RF and power transmission radiation reverse cancer remission? (Question from a patient who was in remission and sent home to a house with power lines over the property—cancer came back very shortly afterwards)

#49. Is it possible to isolate the symptoms and health effects of electromagnetic energy, when we are also being exposed daily to toxins such as pesticides, perchlorate in water, hormones in foods, etc?

#50. Is there a connection between EMF/RF exposure and low thyroid function?

#51. Is there a connection between exponential growth in EMF/RF exposures and the obesity epidemic?

#52. Can you speak to the actual physiological disruption that occurs with exposure— ex: calcium ion mobilization?

#53. Is there a connection between the rise in insulin resistance and EMF exposure?

#54. Is electrical hypersensitivity recognized as a disability?

How to Keep the Body Functioning Optimally in High EMF/RF Environments

#55. Are there any vitamins or natural substances that one can take to reduce EMF sensitivity? (Especially if one already suffers from occasional tremors due to electrical sensitivity)

#56. What can I do to optimize neurological functioning given the daily assaults from these technologies? Are there any proactive steps one can take?

EMF Impact on Drug Absorption

#57. I heard EMF is affecting the efficacy of the breast cancer drug Tamoxifen. Does this suggest it is affecting the efficacy of other pharmaceutical drugs as well?

Health Industry Use of EMF/RF:

#58. What about exposure from X-rays—mammograms, dental x-rays etc?

#59. Is it true frequencies are now being used in research to treat cancer?

#60. Are hospital environments safe for patients from an EMF perspective?

Environmental Health

EMF Impact on Animals & Nature

#61. Have any of you done research on the effect of microwave radiation on bees?

#62. Is it true that birds are dropping out of the sky by the millions due to EMF? Are environmental organizations on to this issue yet?

Measuring Exposures & Exposure Standards

Measuring EMF/RF

#63. Are there tools to measure the amount of EMFs or microwaves in our environment?

#64. What are people called who have these skills? Would an electrician be equipped to assess the EMF/RF environment?

#65. Are there reliable meters for measuring RF?

Exposure Standards & Issues

#66. Is it true that Austria and Russia have far more protective standards? Is this what the US should emulate?

#67. We are currently revising the code for antennas in Richmond, CA. We are asking for a buffer of 1,000 feet from the new higher-powered antennas. Can you advise on a reasonable buffer zone for schools/homes?

Real Estate Related

Real Estate Valuation Impact

#68. How do you know where the antennas are in your neighborhood? Will close proximity to towers devalue property?

Public's Right to Know Whereabouts of Towers/Antennas

#69. Is there anything being done to identify to the public the buildings with cell phone towers on the premises?

#70. Also, what is the law regarding access to roofs with towers? (Question was from a telecom installer)

#71. As a potential renter, or a purchaser of residential property, is disclosure required if there is cell phone equipment in or on or near the building? If not, what are the necessary steps to make this a requirement?

Neighborhood Health Surveys

#72. I live within 300 feet from a cell tower and want to conduct an epidemiological survey of my neighborhood. Are there any resources to help me with this?

Science and Research Related

Research Issues

#73. Why are all current studies of brain tumors from cell phone use funded by the cell phone industry?

#74. Has the US government taken any interest in the BioInitiative Report?

Interphone Study

#75. What exactly is the Interphone Study and is it true the results have been delayed for years?

Dirty Power

#76. What is 'power quality'? And what is 'dirty power'?

#77. Is the source of dirty power exclusively from RF emitting towers and RF emitting consumer products? Did the problem of dirty power exist prior to the cell phone industry?

#78. If I do not use a cell phone or any RF personal equipment, like a cell phone or portable phone, how serious is the impact on my electrical wiring from dirty power?

Science Re. 'Information Carrying Radio Waves'

#79. Can you explain more about why information carrying radio waves are different from regular waves? I want to defend this to my scientifically-minded friends who ridicule the idea.

Satellites

#80. Does radiation from satellites pose similar dangers, or is it too weak?

Underground Power Lines

#81. Are underground power lines as dangerous to our health?

Ground Current

#82. I hear that the utilities are using the earth to return electrical currents to substations instead of returning the currents via neutral wiring. Are there health consequences?

Big Picture

Responsibility for Current RF State of Affairs

#83. Who was responsible for getting Sec. 704 into the Telecommunications Act of 1996, which disallows state and local governments the right to influence the siting of towers on health/environmental grounds? Individual identities should be brought to light and people held accountable!

Attracting Media Coverage of this Issue

#84. I saw an article about cell phone use adding to commute time. Why are journalists not covering the serious health effects also? How can people help to make this FRONT PAGE news?

#85. You said youngsters using cell phones are at greatest risk—are you thinking about engaging the entertainment industry to reach kids? PSA on MTV of P. Diddy or Quincy Jones? Have you done outreach to engage popular icons?

#86. What efforts were made to the national media so they could publicize the BioInitiative Report?

Consequences of Necessary Health-Protecting Changes for Industry and Consumers

#87. If the exposure standards are strengthened, what will be the effect on the communications technology industry? Will there be any reduction of services as a result?

#88. How would we function—and compete—if we do away with wireless appliances?

#89. Is fiber optic technology a viable alternative to Wi-Fi and are there any health consequences with fiber?

#90. Is cable, combined with Wi-Fi into the home, safe?

#91. Has anybody looked at the psychological impact of the invasion of wireless technologies in our lives?

#92.   So, if cell phones are really this bad, what are the alternatives? Is it realistic to believe that all Americans would be willing to give up their cells, blackberries, iPhones, wireless, etc?

#93.   What might be corporate interests in NOT setting protective limits?

#94.   Nearby Radar Station: There is an old navy radar station operating on Mt. Tam in Marin left from the Cold War era which scans the coast and operates 24/7. How much risk does it pose to health if you live in a home and can see Mt. Tam?

Exposure Standards Abroad

#95. Are the governmental standards in Europe and elsewhere more stringent than those in the U.S.? Are the acceptable levels for microwave, RF, etc. in the US higher than in Europe?

#96.   What precautionary steps have been taken abroad on this issue?

BioInitiative Report

#97.   Where can we find a summary of the BioInitiative Report to provide to our City Council?

#98.   Why are the results of the BioInitiative Report so different from the WHO's results? Isn't the output from a cell tower transmitter 50'-150' in the air comparable with output from over the air TV signals?

#99.   What has been the response of the EU and Germany?

Cell Phone Industry Response

#100. Do cell phone manufacturers or service providers acknowledge any health effects? Has anyone checked SEC 10k filings?

#101. What is the importance of the SAR value in assessing cell phone health risks? Why isn't this value available on the box so one can know it before purchasing?

#102. How could the entire industry pretend there are only thermal effects—and get away with it for so long?

Advocacy for Change

#103. Is there an organized effort to amend the portion of the Telecom Act of 1996 that forbids consideration of health and environmental factors when placing towers?

#104. What are the roles of the EPA, FDA, FCC and other federal government agencies with respect to protecting the public from the possible adverse effects of radiofrequency radiation? In other words, who is protecting us?

New Technologies on the Horizon

#105. I hear long-distance Wi-Fi is coming soon, or 'Wi-Max'. It will blanket geographic areas for miles. What can we do *if we don't want this*? It seems to me this will put many sensitive people in jeopardy and contribute to the growth in the electrohypersensitive population. Who is looking out for our health?

#106. What is 'Broadband Over Power' and is this something we should be concerned about? Does it mean radiofrequency radiation transmitted over the electrical wiring?

#107. What are "smart meters" and do they pose a health threat. Can we opt out of using smart meters?

Corporate Social Responsibility

#108. Has there been any outreach to educate corporations through the 'Corporate Social Responsibility' and 'Sustainability in Business' communities?

Legal Possibilities

#109. Halifax, VA became the 1st Virginia town to ban chemical and radioactive bodily trespass, stripping corporations of 'rights', announced 2/7/08. Community Environmental Legal Defense Fund Project Director, Ben Price, said "The people of the town of Halifax have determined that they do not consent to be irradiated, nor to be trespassed upon, by toxic substances that would be released by Virginia Uranium, Inc. or any other state chartered corporation. The people have asserted their right and their duty to protect their families, environment, and future generations. In enacting this law, the community has gone on record as rejecting Dillon's Rule, which erroneously asserts that there is no inherent right to local self government. The American Revolution was about nothing less than the fundamental right of the people to be the decision-makers on issues directly affecting the communities in which they live...The people of Town of Halifax have acted in the best tradition of liberty and freedom, and confronted injustice in the form of a state-permitted corporate assault against the consent of the sovereign people". Doesn't it seem that this approach is needed to protect us from the Telecom corporations?

#110. What can we as citizens do to restore state and local governments' rights to decide if we should be blanketed in wireless technologies? It seems like we don't have a chance anymore for health, and local governments, representing people, need to get involved.

Asked of Audience: How many people in this room have experienced adverse health effects from wireless emissions?

Frequency of Electro-Hypersensitivity Symptoms Based On Distance to Cell Phone Base Station

Electro-Hyper-Sensitivity (EHS)

1. Fatigue *
2. Sleep disturbance *
3. Headaches
4. Feeling of discomfort
5. Difficulty in concentrating *
6. Depression *
7. Memory loss *
8. Visual disruptions *
9. Irritability *
10. Hearing disruptions *
11. Skin problems
12. Cardiovascular *
13. Dizziness *
14. Loss of appetite *
15. Movement of difficulties *
16. Nausea

* Associated with Aging:
"Rapid Aging Syndrome"

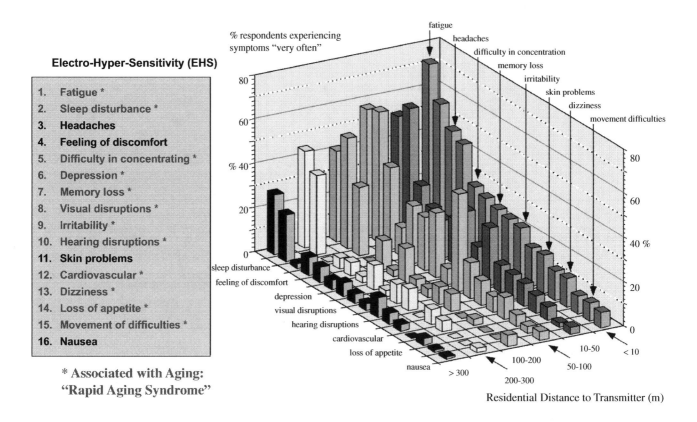

Source: Symptoms experience by people in the vicinity of cellular phone base station, Santini 2001, La Presse Medicale

110 Questions from The Commonwealth Club Audience

We highly recommend readers listen to the panel presentation from which the questions below were generated, found in the Commonwealth Club archives at http://www.commonwealthclub.org/archive/08/08-03microwaveradiation-audio.html or at www.ElectromagneticHealth.org

Personal Safety

Cell Phone & Portable Phone Use & Safety

#1. Is there a safe distance to hold a cell or portable phone away when using its speakerphone?

MH: Scientists don't know if there is a safe distance but most will tell you to hold the phone as far away from your body as possible.

CR: Recent experiments (Salford et al. 2007) show impact on the brain at a distance of more than 1 meter ("Non-thermal Effects of EMF Upon the Mammalian Brain: The Lund Experience", Leif G. Salford et al., The Environmentalist Vol. 27, pg 493-500, 2007). So, if you use a cell phone, use the speakerphone as far away from your body as practically possible.

#2. Are the earpiece phones "safe"?

MH: It is unclear if the question is about using an earpiece (headset) with the cell phone or using a cell phone that attaches directly to your ear.

For the first interpretation (using a wired earpiece with a cell phone): RF is emitted along the length of the cord all the way to your ear. Since the cord is generally touching or close to the body it means that the body is irradiated more with an earpiece than without.

If the question is about phones that attach to the ear then I would suggest these are worse as you do not change the side of the head that you use to talk on the phone, and hence expose one side of the brain to more radiation than if you shifted the phone from side to side.

CR: Note that wireless Bluetooth earpieces with cell phones are believed by many scientists to be more dangerous than cell phones alone, because even though they use much lower power near the head, and radiate lower levels of radiation than cell phones, they are always 'on', and also use wireless technology put right onto or even into your ear.

According to a University of York study http://www.mobiledia.com/news/24586.html (measuring SAR values in a fake human head), as well as a study conducted by Stan Hartman of RadSafe in Boulder, CO (www.radsafe.net), wired headsets do reduce radiation levels significantly at the head, and are therefore probably safer than using the cell phone alone, or than using wireless Bluetooth. The Hartman assessment, measuring raw power levels, found at least a 95% reduction at the head.

Please note, however, that radiation can enter the body anywhere on its surface, not just at the head, so this is not to imply that using cell phones with a wired headset is safe. They simply may be safer from the perspective of direct exposure to the head.

Also, Hartman adds, "There's no way to predict what all phones will do with all headsets without actually testing each model, because how much radiation may be induced in the headset (if any) depends on the design of the particular phone, especially the location of the headset jack in relation to the antenna. I have found a 3-fold difference in radiation levels using different headset brands with the same phone." "However, behind all this," he adds, "is the troubling question of whether it's power levels at all that are the problem, or maybe the frequencies instead, or some combination thereof."

#3. My cordless phone is in my bedroom about 10' from my body when sleeping, is this distance safe?

MH: There are two types of cordless phones. One is a DECT phone that radiates 24/7 and the other is a regular cordless phone that works like a cell phone and radiates ONLY when it is used. The DECT phone should be banned because it is like having a cell phone antenna right in your home. They are powerful and radiation can be picked up in rooms other than the room that contains this phone.

Indeed they can be picked up in neighboring homes as well. The only way to know for sure if your cordless phone is a problem (i.e. a DECT phone) is to have someone measure the radio frequency coming from the phone.

CR: Many health professionals recommend not using DECT (Digital Enhanced Cordless Telecommunications) cordless phones at all, and especially not in the bedroom where one sleeps. Radiofrequency fields cause sleep disruption, deplete key hormones, such as melatonin, and have been associated with a wide range of dysfunctions, including genetic effects, cancer, cardiovascular effects, immune system changes, blood-brain barrier permeability, nervous system disruption, etc. For more information see "Cordless Phones: The Unspoken DECT Hazard at Home and at Work" at http://www.tetrawatch.net/science/dect.php

#4. Do cell and portable phones affect us biologically if they are turned on but not being used?

MH: When cell phones are on standby they emit a periodic pulse to make connection with the nearest antenna. Total radiation exposure of the person is much lower and much shorter in duration in this mode than when the person is talking.

CR: Re. portable cordless phones, see # 3 above. If it is a DECT portable phone it radiates 24/7.

Cell phones also emit very low-frequency magnetic fields due to the battery-conservation system, which are biologically active if near the body, according to Stan Hartman of RadSafe in Boulder, CO. The low frequency magnetic fields from the battery-conserving system in cell phones are in the human brain wave frequency. Please note that The Options Brief of the European Parliament's "The Physiological and Environmental Effects of Non-Ionizing Radiation—Final Study" says that it should be made clear to consumers that "shields and ear pieces afford no protection against the low frequency pulsed magnetic field from the battery of the phone."

#5. Regarding earpieces for cell phones, are wireless receivers even worse than putting the phone to your ear?

MH: A wireless receiver-transmitter has to communicate with the cell phone, which is often fairly close. A cell phone has to communicate with an antenna that might be several miles away. As a result the radiation from the wireless earpiece/ headset to the phone is much lower than from the cell phone to the antenna, however the human being is affected by both.

CR: Note that recent research suggests that lower levels of radiation can sometimes be worse than higher levels. More research on the dose-response relationship, and especially on this paradox, is necessary.

#6. What about Bluetooth headpieces—are they dangerous?

MH: I would suggest using a landline first, a cell phone in speaker mode second and neither a wireless headset nor a wired headset.

#7. Bluetooth headsets are radiating about 1 milligauss. Are they safe?

MH: It isn't so much the magnetic field (which is what milligauss measures) but rather the power density at the head that one needs be concerned about. Both wired earpieces and wireless Bluetooth headsets emit radiation so we need some serious measurements of the relative and absolute power density while using these devices. My answer is that cell phones with wired or wireless headsets are NOT SAFE.

#8. Does it not stand to reason that Bluetooth devices cause cancer as well? Is it not true that the wires in the headsets increase the danger not decrease it?

MH: We did some random measurements and we found that the wired headset radiates along the entire length of the wire. As a result I would not recommend using this type of device unless manufacturers begin to make them with a shielded wire and a pneumatic tube (i.e. air tube) near the ear. The pneumatic tubes are available but I don't know if earpieces with shielded cords are available.

CR: According to the Hartman analysis mentioned above, power levels at the headset earpiece are 95-99% lower than at the phone. Thus while a wire of any kind will pick up and transmit microwave radiation (including a limited amount from stray RF in a typical city environment), he notes "the wire won't be putting out anything like the levels close to a phone". Please recognize however, that while the phone itself, if you are using a headset, will not be near one's brain, it nonetheless will be radiating close to other body parts (e.g. your hand, stomach, kidney, liver, ovaries etc.)

So do not construe the significantly reduced power at the level of the head when using a wired headset to imply using a wired headset is safe. Also recognize that other metal objects in one's personal environment, beyond the wire to the headset, such as eye glasses, underwire bras, metal bed coils, jewelry, metal furniture, IUDs, metal fillings in your teeth, or braces, etc. may create hazardous hotspots, increasing your exposure.

#9. How much effect does an ear phone have on the health effects of cell phones?

MH: Anything that reduces a person's exposure to radiation will reduce their risk of cancer and other health problems. Hence using a phone less, less often, for shorter periods, shifting phone from ear to ear (this will reduce exposure to one side of the head), not using phone when reception is bad and it is roaming (since levels of radiation are much higher at this time) are ways of reducing your exposure. If someone is serious about reducing adverse health effects of a cell phone they should use a cell phone ONLY in circumstances when other options of communication are unavailable. Those who have given up landlines and use only cell phones today should be told the prudent thing to do is to re-install a landline.

CR: Wired headsets do dramatically reduce exposure at the head, if the phone is kept away from the body. People who need to use a cell phone while traveling will often use the phone with a headset and then attach an extension cord to assure the phone remains at a significant distance from the physical body. Otherwise, the phone remains near waist level or in a pocket or on a belt holster where radiation exposure to abdominal organs is still occurring and dissipating internal to the body.

#10. What is more dangerous—the power or the frequencies of cell phones, or both?

MH: Both the intensity (power) and frequency (GHz and lower frequencies) are likely to be important. We simply don't know the relative effects of these. Also important to consider are characteristics such as modulation, waveform, bandwidth, peakpower, pulsed vs. continuous wave, pulse width and duty cycle.

CR: Heat shock proteins in cells occur at levels way lower than the heating effect from the 'power' exposure (See Bioelectromagnetics, 2004 Dec; 25(8): 642-6; discussion 647-8, "A Biological Guide for Electromagnetic Safety: The Stress Response", M. Blank, R. Goodman), indicating cells are indeed being stressed by the invisible glare of electromagnetic radiation. See also Health and Stress, The Newsletter of the American Institute of Stress, Number 6, 2008, "Stress, Cell Phones and Electro-Smog".

'Protection' Devices—Do They Work?

#11. Do the small devices people attach to cell and cordless phones actually cut the EMF levels to a 'safe' limit?

MH: I don't know. I haven't seen any credible scientific studies conducted by independent researchers. Also we haven't been able to measure any changes in radiation. However, some people swear by them while others don't notice anything. We need well-conducted studies to answer this question.

CR: Some scientists believe that, at best, these device mask symptoms (sometimes by altering brain waves). Please note there is little evidence to date showing they prevent types of injury known to be occurring (injury to DNA, cell membranes, blood vessels, blood cells, brain cells, nerves, heart, thyroid, adrenals, etc, even if people feel improved using them. One study, however, does show bioprotection of cellular and systemic stress from cell phones via emission of an ultra-weak compensatory field (Journal of Cellular Biochemistry. Vol. 89, Issue 1, 2003.pages 48-55, by Weisbrot, Lin, Ye, Blank and Goodman).

While there is no change in radiation exposure, and as of yet no evidence of change in damage to the body on most of the above parameters, there are a few parties working with 'subtle energy' who have demonstrated reduction of cell phone radiation's impact on the autonomic nervous system, as measured by heart rate variability (HRV) devices and other measures. Research is ongoing and has not as of yet been published. Check·back at ElectromagneticHealth.org for updates.

#12. I have seen body pendants and whole house blockers of radiation. Are these legitimately helpful?

MH: See answer above. Some electrically sensitive people who have tried various pendants have noticed some benefits that eventually wear off. Others felt worse wearing them, and some don't notice any difference. I would simply say, "buyer beware". Perhaps the government agencies that test claims made by companies should do their job and test these devices, especially the ones that make medical claims.

CR: I used one such pendant for many months. When it was misplaced, symptoms of electrical hypersensitivity became much worse than they had been in the first place. I learned from this experience I don't want to be dependent on something external to myself to function well, and that the better strategy is to clean up one's home and office environments of EMFs so one doesn't need to attempt to manipulate one's physiological functioning in this way.

Note also that using this pendant allowed me to stay in a very high EMF environment months longer than I should have, and it permitted me to easily deceive myself that I was 'safe' when in fact I was not. My apartment building had installed a wireless internet system throughout, frequencies from a neighbor's wireless router were coming through the wall into my bedroom and the building was in the vicinity of 941 cell phone antennas (a number that one and a half years later has grown—unknown to residents—to over 1,300). The public's #1 focus should be on 1) changing EMF exposure standards at the federal level, and 2) giving state and local governments back the right to limit the proliferation of wireless technologies in their communities, not on finding ways to live in higher and higher EMF environments using pendants and the like.

Consumers should also beware that many pendants marketed today are said by users and people who have evaluated them to have no effect whatsoever. These products are unregulated and generally untested by independent laboratories.

#13. Is there any product out there that we could use to protect us from EMR—for example, Teslar watches?

MH: See answer above.

#14. Do you have any comment on WillauTronic products—esmog protection with transponder chip technology for cell phones, TVs, microwave ovens, cordless phones, etc? Or BioPro, Aegisguard, etc?

MH: I'm not familiar with these technologies. See comments above re. need to address federal level policy issues.

CR: Hartman notes that only some kinds of shielding material, like Microshield or Skin-Blok, will reduce exposure to microwaves, but note not from the phone's ELF magnetic fields. These fields can be very harmful, especially in the case of Blackberries and other PDAs, etc. (Jokela et al. 2004; Sage et al. 2007). See "Personal Digital Assistant (PDA) Cell Phone Units

Produce Elevated Extremely-Low Frequency Electromagnetic Field Emissions" by C. Sage, O. Johansson and S. Amy Sage at http://www.buergerwelle.de/pdf/sage_pda_bems_on_line.pdf

For Safety Resources used by leading EMF environmental consultants, please go to www.EMFSafetyStore.com.

Home Health re. EMF/RF

#15. Are we more vulnerable while sleeping?

MH: Yes. Sleep is a period of regeneration. If this process is interfered with it can have adverse effects. Also during sleep our production of melatonin increases. High levels of melatonin seem to protect us against various types of cancer, including breast cancer. Light at night as well as exposure to other frequencies of electromagnetic energy reduces melatonin production, which may interfere with our body's ability to fight cancer.

CR: Also note that cell phone usage during the day has been shown to alter sleep patterns at night. Sleep is often one of the first things affected in people of all ages. According to Deitrich Klinghardt MD, PhD we are hundreds of times more sensitive during sleep. He recommends shutting off fuses at night (or installing a "demand switch" near your bed), replacing cordless phones with corded phones, and having no wireless internet. Extremely sensitive people, as well as high performance athletes, and savvy executives who travel extensively, sleep under metal mesh tents that block out microwaves.

#16. Can you tell us about the risk and distance factors for having a Wi-Fi router or are you saying Wi-Fi is too dangerous to have in a house at all?

MH: If you don't want to live near an antenna then why put one inside your home? A wireless router is like a mini antenna. Use a hard-wired router, just as hard-wired telephones, in all cases.

CR: According to environmental consultant Stan Hartman in Boulder, CO, when people have Wi-Fi antennas in a router on their desks, they are getting about the same amount of radiation as they would 30 meters or less from the large outdoor antennas of a typical cell phone base station (though the Wi-Fi signal typically isn't as constant as a cell signal). He says people should put the wireless router as far away from occupied areas as possible to still get a signal, if they choose to use Wi-Fi at all. Note also that if one has the computer off, but the router still on, one is still being subject to frequencies from the router as it pulses periodically looking to make a connection. So make sure to turn the router off when it is not in use. Hartman says, "One reason Wi-Fi (and cordless phones) can be more dangerous even than cell phones is because it transmits at full power, rather than having a 'smart system' like a phone does that uses only as much transmitting power as it needs at a given time. Wi-Fi is also often 'on' 24/7, not giving the body any break, and also note there is evidence that non-ionizing radiation has a cumulative effect, like ionizing radiation (see Question #17, following). So, like with lead and mercury, and radioactivity, in a sense there are no safe levels—when you turn off the exposure to Wi-Fi the living system doesn't go back to the way it was but remains somewhat damaged."

Hartman says, "If Alasdair Phillips of Power Watch (www.powerwatch.org.uk) is right about health effects beginning at about 0.001 µW/cm2 (and I think that's generous, especially for electrosensitives), Wi-Fi in the same room is exposing people to at least 30 times bioactive levels."

Citywide Wi-Fi, or the super high power Wi-Max coming our way very soon, is thus a matter of very serious health concern, not only for the health of humans but for animals and nature as well. With 24/7 Wi-Fi systems, there is no down time to rebalance from the electromagnetic interference with the body. Congress should urgently reevaluate Wi-Max approvals before it is too late.

#17. What evidence is there for cumulative effects of microwave radiation from cell phones and Wi-Fi?

CR: See "Neurological Effects of Radiofrequency Radiation" by Henry Lai, PhD, Bioelectromagnetics Research Laboratory, Department of Bioengineering, School of Medicine and College of Engineering, University of Washington, (http://www.mapcruzin.com/radiofrequency/henry_lai2.htm): "...results indicate changes in the response characteristics of the nervous system with repeated exposure, suggesting that the effects are not 'forgotten' after each episode of exposure."

According to Lucinda Grant, author of Microwave Sickness, the Soviets were particularly concerned about the cumulative effects of non-thermal radiation doses, including reproductive and genetic effects." Her references were Baranski, S. and P. Czerski, Biological Effects of Microwaves, 1976; Gordon, Z.V., ed. Biological Effects of Radiofrequency Electromagnetic Fields, U.S. Joint Publications Research Service, 1974 and Biologic Effects and Health Hazards of Microwave Radiation, Polish Medical Publishers, 1974. (http://omega.twoday.net/stories/314911/)

See also "Biological Effects of Radiofrequency Radiation" by Wolfgang W. Scherer (http://www.reach.net/~scherer/p/biofx.htm), in which he discusses the accumulation of RF damage in eyes:

"What distinguishes radiofrequency introduced heating from other means of heating is the rapidity of heating, the depth of penetration, and the existence of internal hot-spots, that can result in tissue damage long before the overall body temperature increases dramatically.

The brain is particularly susceptible to the occurrence of these hot-spots. Depending on the size of the head and the frequency of the radiation, regions of relatively high absorption can occur at or near the center of the brain. These effects are especially uncontrollable in the near-field during the use of mobile communication devices like cordless and cellular phones and very unpredictable due to the variable shape, size, and thickness of skulls.

"However, the main objectively measurable hazard of microwave radiation is injury to the eyes, especially damaging at frequencies above 800 MHz. Since the lens of the eye does not have an adequate vascular system for the exchange of heat, even a slight rise in temperature can cause protein coagulation, and opacities in the lens may form."

Finally, chronic health conditions linked to EMF should also be considered. For a brief summary, please see "Microwave and Radiofrequency Radiation Exposure: A Growing Environmental Health Crisis" by Cindy Sage, located on the San Francisco Medical Society's website at http://www.sfms.org/AM/Template.cfm?Section=Home&CONTENTID=1770&TEM PLATE=/C M/HTMLDisplay.cfm&SECTION=Article_Archive

Here you will find a list of EMF related symptoms and conditions, and start to understand the extraordinary toll unchecked electromagnetic radiation exposure is having on our health care system and health costs. These include "changes in cell membrane function, major changes in calcium metabolism and cellular signal communication, cell proliferation, activation of proto-oncogenes, activation of HSP heat shock proteins as if heating has occurred when it has not, and cell death. Resulting effects reported in the scientific literature include DNA breaks and chromosome aberrations, increased free radical production, cell stress and premature aging, changes in brain function including memory loss, learning impairment, headaches and fatigue, sleep disorders, neurodegenerative conditions, reduction in melatonin secretion and cancer."

#18. Is there any risk standing near a microwave oven when it is operating? What distance?

MH: Yes. I recommend that you leave the kitchen when the microwave oven is on. Every single microwave oven that I have measured leaks microwaves. One way that you can test your microwave oven for leakage is to put your cell phone inside the oven (but do NOT turn the oven on). If you then call your phone and it rings, the signal had to pass through the walls of the microwave oven. This is a reliable test only if you are able to get a cell phone signal in your kitchen.

CR: Microwave ovens are allowed by U.S. law to leak as much as 5 mW/cm^2. According to environmental consultant Stan Hartman, "They also put out HUGE ELF magnetic fields – comparable to the fields from garbage disposals – and the control panels usually have very strong ELF magnetic fields around them (100 mG or more at the surface is common), even when the oven is off but plugged in." People sensitive to RF/ELF should take note.

At 4 mG or more, studies have shown risk of childhood leukemia doubles. And with exposure at 16 mG, a Kaiser Permanente epidemiological study found an up to six-fold increased risk of spontaneous abortions among pregnant women. (Li, D-K, R. Odoull, S. Wi, T. Janevic, I. Golditch, T.D. Bracken, R. Senior, R. Rankin, and R. Iriye. 2002, *"A population-based perspective cohort study of personal exposure to magnetic fields during pregnancy and the risk of miscarriage."* Epidemiology 13:9-20.)

The above should make clear the importance of staying away from the high ELF magnetic fields of microwave ovens, as well as from the radiofrequency fields being emitted.

#19. A friend uses a microwave with a cracked glass door, I told her not to, can you confirm the danger?

MH: **It is both dangerous and stupid!**

CR: Like many cognitively impaired people today, this person's level of consciousness, presence, and awareness of the fragile dimensions of living systems appears to be low.

#20. What are the health effects of microwave ovens?

MH: **Microwave ovens use similar frequencies to cell phones and mobile phones. These microwaves are selectively absorbed by water and fat. Eyes are very sensitive to these frequencies and there is an increased likelihood of developing cataracts. Hence it is important not to stand in front of a microwave oven to watch your food heating. Ideally you should leave the kitchen when microwave is on. See also Question #18 re. magnetic fields.**

CR: Note some believe there may also be physiological effects from consuming microwaved food, but this is not an area with which we are familiar. There has been very little formal research in this area.

#21. Are energy efficient bulbs (i.e. Compact Fluorescent Bulbs) actually bad for our living space? Please elucidate.

MH: **YES!**

These bulbs contain mercury and this mercury is released into the environment when the bulb is broken, burnt or dumped at a landfill site.

Compact fluorescent lights (CFLs) generate ultraviolet radiation (UV), which may exacerbate skin problems according to Philippe Laroche, Media Relations Officer for Health Canada (2008).

CFLs generate RF radiation through the air and may interfere with other types of wireless technology transmitting at similar frequencies.

Most CFLs and tube fluorescent lights (TFL) produce 'dirty electricity', which travels along the wiring in your house and affects people who are electrically sensitive.

An energy efficient alternative to CFL bulbs is LEDs (light emitting diodes). LEDs are much more energy efficient than CFLs and do not contain mercury or generate RF. LEDs that have transformers generate dirty electricity and are not recommended unless filters are used to mop up the dirty electricity. CLEDs do not generate dirty power and are the best lights available on the market from both a health and an environmental perspective.

Note that incandescent lights are also clean electromagnetically but are not energy efficient. Any light that produces heat is inefficient. Some CFLs also produce considerable heat and are not as energy efficient as some think.

CR: At this point the cleanest CLED manufacturer we have found has CLED replacements for fluorescent tubes, halogen bulbs and direct task lamp lighting, but not a CLED bulb yet to replace the standard incandescent bulb. Minimum orders, shipped from Asia, are 1,000 units. If you are a distributor, let us know if we can put you in touch.

#22. What is a safe level of EMF/RF to live with?

MH: We don't know what levels are "safe" but we do know the lower the better. For constant exposure to (1) Extremely Low Frequency *Magnetic* Field should be below 1 mG (although ambient levels are generally around 0.1 to 0.2 mG or lower; (2) Extremely Low Frequency *Electric* Field ideally below 5 V/m; (3) For constant exposure to Radio Frequency Radiation (RFR), the best guidelines so far are the Salzburg guidelines at 1000 microwatts/m² (0.1 microWatts/cm²), however, electrically sensitive people react to MUCH lower levels of RFR; and (4) Dirty electricity below 40 GS units. While these levels may be "safe" for most people, those who have become electrically sensitive may have difficulty at these exposures.

CR: A document entitled Radio Wave Packet contains charts of key research for your reference, some dating as far back as 1950. It lists biological effects of radiowaves at different power densities, international exposure standards, select clinical studies of workers exposed on the job and epidemiological studies. http://www.goodhealthinfo.net/radiation/radio_wave_packet.pdf

#23. Does having solar panels on a roof cause problems?

MH: Solar panels use DC/AC converters that produce dirty electricity, which has adverse health effects. See Question #27 which mentions some of the known health effects of dirty electricity as well as the section on Dirty Power beginning with Question #76. Many houses with solar panels have very high dirty electricity.

CR: This is one of many examples of the 'green' and 'sustainability' movements promoting technologies or products as preferable, when they may offer energy efficiencies but at the same time also have very negative effects on human health.

#24. Where do we get the filters to eliminate 'dirty electricity' on home and office wiring created by high RF environments? Are these considered legitimate as compared to the controversy around pendants that claim to be protective?

MH: www.stetzerelectric.com. We've tested these filters in U.S schools and we found that about 35% of the teachers noticed significant improvements in their health/well being.

It is important to realize that these filters are designed to improve power quality and have no effect on RF coming through the air. Not everyone who uses them will notice improvements. Electrical sensitivity is a very complex issue that requires a lot more research. Sensitive individuals can usually tell if they notice a difference or not. If you make any change, assess what you notice and follow your instincts to determine if this is a worthwhile strategy.

#25. Are TV remotes ELF transmitters?

MH: Some use infrared energy. Infrared is at a different frequency than RF. Infrared doesn't interfere with radio frequency communication and is presumed to be safe as it is used in such things as infrared saunas.

CR: No TV remotes I know of, including the rare RF remotes, are ELF transmitters but all do emit infrared pulses when transmitting an infrared signal (i.e. *while pressing the buttons*).

Some people are also sensitive to infrared, some even more so than microwave radiation. There is research showing individuals with porphyrin enzyme deficiency (associated with electrohypersensitivity) can be specifically sensitive to infrared frequencies.

#26. Can bed springs conduct these frequencies? What about metal furniture?

MH: Yes. Anything metal can reradiate these frequencies. Including all metal furniture. One especially should minimize metal furniture in the bedroom, or in an office where one spends long hours.

#27. What's the problem with plasma TVs?

MH: Plasma TVs generate very high levels of dirty electricity and a number of scientific peer-reviewed studies show that dirty electricity has adverse health effects. Some documented health effects of dirty electricity include difficulty sleeping, chronic fatigue, chronic pain, neurological disorders, skin problems, difficulty thinking clearly and problems with short-term memory, nausea, ringing in the ears, etc.

#28. Where would we find the reflecting fabric? Does this protect from microwave radiation as well as from dirty electricity? Are there circumstances when it should not be used?

MH: You can get RF reflecting fabric at www.safelivingtechnologies.ca or www. EMFSafetyStore.com. It reflects analogue and pulsed digital radio frequency (RF) waves from sources such as microwave, Wi-Fi, and cell phone towers. The best product has the densest weave.

It works optimally in the 0.2 to 10 GHz range and is much less effective at shielding dirty electricity, which is in the kHz range. One must be careful using reflecting fabric and first be informed by actual RF measurements so one is certain from what directions the RF is coming. For example, one wouldn't want to put up the fabric on all 4 walls while using a computer or other RF emitting technology within, as the effects would be to increase a person's exposure. Its best to hire an environmental consultant trained in Electromagnetic Fields rather than try to guess how to use these fabrics.

CR: Worth noting is that some competitive athletes sleep under protective tents at night for optimal repair and regeneration, as do many electrically sensitive people, and increasingly, savvy executives. There are also shielding paints on the market though these require grounding procedures and their use is still controversial. Always work with a professional environmental consultant trained in EMF.

After all is said and done, remember how important it is to be connected to the natural fields coming from the earth. Getting outside in nature is more important now than ever!

#29. Do you have any help to offer those of us fighting the installation of antenna towers (and labeled crazies)?

MH: EMR Policy Institute in Vermont www.EMRPolicy.org; Council on Wireless Technology Impacts www.energyfields.org in California; www.weepinitiative.ca in Canada; and www.hese.uk in UK. A good strategy always is to talk with people in communities that have been successful and these groups help you make these connections.

CR: The telecom infrastructure will continue to be built-out until consumers get involved and say 'Enough!' This means being heard by government officials, as well as taking a stand with one's pocketbook by not buying into the fallacy that we need these technologies, and that they improve our quality of life, when in many ways they take away from quality of life, impair our health and often are not necessary.

Recently the town of Richmond Hill in Canada unanimously turned down an application from Rogers Wireless to build a tower after residents protested. Residents insisted they did not want the 'better service'. In the US it is hard to win fights against cell towers—all the more reason for people to raise their voices louder, together, taking a stand for our individual and collective Electromagnetic Health. I suggest **everyone sign the Petition to Congress found at www.ElectromagneticHealth.org and also write your Congress person and ask him or her to read *"Public Health SOS: The Shadow Side of the Wireless Revolution"*** so they better understand EMF effects on humans, animals and nature and become engaged with this issue. Also see, "Cell Towers, Wireless Convenience? Or Environmental Hazard?" edited by B. Blake Levitt (Safe Goods/New Century, 2001), for valuable information re. tower siting issues.

#30. How far away do cell phone towers have to be from your home to be 100% safe?

MH: It is impossible to be 100% safe. Studies show adverse health associations for people who live within 400 meters (0.24 miles) of cell phone antennas and 2 Km (1.2 miles) from broadcast antennas. However, it should be remembered that "distance" is a surrogate for "power density" (or the strength of the radiation) and it is not a particularly good surrogate as all sorts of things can increase or decrease the strength of the radiation. See information below.

CR: People who are electrically sensitive can often feel effects from some cell towers 2- 3 miles away. It is imperative people take into consideration the power of the antenna(s). In Golden, CO, for example, there is a tower whose television and other antennas put out about 1 million watts, and the dangerous effects can be measured more than 5 miles away (there's also a 10 million watt facility planned). Note also that one can be close to an antenna as the crow flies, but with a mountain in between, where you wouldn't be affected at all. So it is hard to generalize. One must take measurements to know the exposure levels for sure.

Also recognize that the power levels coming from antennas on a nearby cell tower could be increased at any time without your knowledge.

Stan Hartman, an environmental consultant experienced in measuring EMF, adds, "It's difficult to generalize about safe distances from cell towers. Putting aside the variables that have to do with personal health, personal genetic profile and so forth, there are also landscape factors to consider – weather, humidity, how many obstructions are between the tower and the subject, what their geometry is, what they're composed of. Then there are the questions of how many antennas are on the tower; their geometry, angle, and beam pattern; the level of cell traffic the tower is serving, how far away the traffic is, the angle of the antennas, etc.

"What I'm saying is that you *really need to measure to know exposure levels* for sure, and with more than a single-time test. There should probably be 24-hr. measurements over several days, keeping in mind that the radiation levels could change over time as more traffic is added or removed.

"It is also possible that being very close to the antenna could offer less exposure than farther away, especially if there are good microwave insulators intervening, like brick or concrete walls for absorption, or metal or other conductors for reflection.

"If the subject has a clear line of site relationship with the antennas, they will of course be more exposed for a given distance—though again that depends on the beam pattern.

"In a single test of some antennas near our local homeless shelter in Boulder, CO, across an open parking lot, levels about 20 yards from the array (which were situated about 25 feet off the ground on a building) were about 3100 nW/cm^2 (3.4 V/m)—less both closer to and farther from the source. Levels at the near wall of the shelter (outside, about 100 yards away) were about 500 nW/cm^2 (1.4 V/m). A mile away across some neighborhoods of one- and two-story homes, a lake, and some open space, levels are less than 0.05 nW/cm^2 (14 mV/m), but I have no way to tell if these low levels are coming from that antenna array. On top of a hill about a mile away, with a clear line-of-sight to the antennas, levels are 9-10 nW/cm^2 (180-190 mV/m).

"It's very difficult to accurately measure exposure levels in urban or suburban environments at any distance more than a few hundred yards, because of the profusion of sources and reflections. Even with a directional antenna, you don't know if you're picking up a primary signal or a reflection.

"Based on these readings, and with the caveats above, I'd say that if you're one kilometer away in an urban or suburban environment you're probably in the 'safe' zone, but that distance these days will probably put you closer to other microwave sources. There really isn't any way to generalize and answer the question just in terms of distance."

#31. What are you the panelists doing to reduce your own and your families' exposures to these hazards?

MH: Dirty Electricity: Installed Graham Stetzer (GS) filters. I use incandescent bulbs and CLEDs but NOT Compact Fluorescents (CFL) in my home. I have an LCD TV and not a plasma TV.

ELF: Bought home far from power lines and transformers. I moved my clock radio away from the head of my bed. I do not use a waterbed or electric blanket and seldom use a hair dryer.

RFR: I bought a home far from antennas and I do not have wireless technology in my home except for one cordless phone that is NOT a DECT phone. I use my cell phone infrequently and only for critical phone calls when I am traveling.

CR: Moved from a high EMF city to a lower EMF region. Live in a house, not an apartment building where one is easily subject to RF from neighbors. Minimal use of cell phone, and only when traveling. Don't use cell phone when traveling in remote areas because of the excess power needed for connection in remote areas. Never leave cell phone turned on and discourage others from calling. Stopped using cordless phones. Stay away from large stores with wireless, and electronics stores.

Avoid Wi-Fi cafes. Seek out hotels with hard-wired computer connections, not Wi-Fi. Studying RF/ELF measurement so I can rely on myself to assess environments. Investing in measurement equipment, and have RF shielding film on the windows of my office. There are so few people trained in remediation in the U.S. it is essential to be self-sufficient! My hope is for every community to send someone for training to assess and remediate electromagnetic fields. Health practitioners might want to attend the Institute for Neurobiology's EMF conference held annually in Seattle so they can competently advise their patients (www.klinghardtneurobiology.com).

#32. Within months of installing a wireless internet network and wireless audio system in our house, mold developed. Is there any connection between wireless and mold?

CR: In a Collaborative for Health and the Environment "EMF Working Group" post, several research references were provided showing a potential RF link with mold (see below). A review is also underway of several multi-million dollar mold lawsuits, finding RF issues, such as antenna farms on roofs or nearby, were potentially important overlooked factors. The connection with mold deserves more investigation, particularly due to the increased amount of mold-related health problems in the U.S. over the past decade.

Some mold references:

Z Naturforsch. 1978 Jan-Feb;33(1-2):15-22. "Nonthermal Effects of Millimeter Microwaves on Yeast Growth"; Grundler W, Keilmann F.

J Microw Power. 1979 Dec;14(4):307-12. "Determination of a Thermal Equivalent of Millimeter Microwaves in Living Cells"; Dardalhon M, Averbeck D, Berteaud AJ.

J Microw Power. 1980 Jun;15(2):75-80. "Response of Aspergillus nidulans and Physarum Polycephalum to Microwave Irradiation"; Mezykowski T, Bal J, Debiec H, Kwarecki K.

Z Naturforsch. 1989 Sep-Oct;44(9-10):863-6. "Resonant Microwave Effect on Locally Fixed Yeast Microcolonies"; Grundler W, Keilmann F.

Bioelectrochem Bioenerg. 1999 Feb;48(1):177-80. "The Effects of Radiofrequency Fields on Cell Proliferation are Non-Thermal"; Velizarov S, Raskmark P, Kwee S.

Phys Med Biol. 2002 Nov 7;47(21):3831-9. "Preliminary Results on the Non-Thermal Effects of 200-350 GHz Radiation on the Growth Rate of S. Cerevisiae Cells in Microcolonies"; Hadjiloucas S, Chahal MS, Bowen JW.

Mikrobiol Z. 2004 May-Jun;66(3):51-7. [Effect of Radio-Frequency Electromagnetic Radiation on Physiological Features of Saccharomyces Cerevisiae Strain UCM Y-517][Article in Russian]; Voĭchuk SI, Podgorskiĭ VS, Gromozova EN.

Finally, in a study with which Deitrich Klinghardt, MD, PhD was involved, mold was grown in a faraday cage blocking out EMFs. When the faraday cage was taken away the amount of neurotoxins generated by the mold increased 600x. He cautions that in the presence of EMFs, it appears the stress on the mold steps up neurotoxin production dramatically.

#33. Do batteries emit less radiation than, say, electrical cords?

MH: If you plug a computer into the wall socket it is using alternating current. If you run the computer on battery it is using direct current. Most, but not all, electrically sensitive people are better able to tolerate battery-operated computers than computers plugged into the wall.

CR: According to Stan Hartman of RadSafe in Boulder, while batteries emit no radiation per se, they do have a very low-voltage static electric field, and when current is actually flowing from one terminal to another, a static magnetic field.

The equipment that the batteries are energizing, though, can emit all kinds of radiation, for example with walkie-talkies, PDAs, cell phones, etc. For example, a computer can have AC magnetic and electric fields and microwaves coming out of it even if battery powered.

Automobiles

#34. Are cars equipped with Blue Tooth especially toxic?

MH: I don't know.

CR: Note that using a cell phone while driving uses more power as the phone must continually be reconnecting with antennas while moving. Also, using a phone while in a car has to put out more signal to get out of the metal and windows, and the radiation is also amplified by internal reflections in the car. It is best not to use any kind of wireless radiation in a car, and if you must use it, use it holding the phone out an open window (while the car is stopped).

Please note that 45 countries now ban cell phone use while driving (http://www.cellularnews.com/car_bans/). In the UK and Wales, people now risk a prison sentence for driving impaired by a cell phone. It is best not to use wireless phones in automobiles.

#35. Are hybrid cars dangerous for our health? What levels of EMF exposure compared to non-hybrids?

MH: Hybrid cars can have high magnetic fields especially near the battery, which tends to be behind the back seat, but not to such a degree one would want to avoid hybrid cars unless one is electrically sensitive. See the Hartman analysis mentioned below. Electrically sensitive people, as long as they are not chemically sensitive, prefer diesel cars because they don't use spark plugs.

CR: See recent *New York Times* article 4/27/08 *"Hybrid Risk Still Uncertain"*. A recent analysis on a Prius hybrid using many measuring tools was done by Stan Hartman of RadSafe in Boulder, CO. He says misunderstandings about measurements with the "frequency-weighted" Trifield meter, which reads high frequencies as high magnetic fields, have led people to believe hybrid cars are far worse for health than they are, as suggested by the NYT article. Magnetic field levels on the back seat peak at 6-8 mG, according to Hartman, but only on hard acceleration, and at other times they average about 3 mG. "At head height and on the front seats they were much lower, and comparable to background levels in the average home. The Trifield meter literature explains the limitations for magnetic field measurements in high frequency environments, but this evidently was not taken into consideration by those who get false 100 mG readings in the hybrid car." Hartman says "I'd hate to see people avoiding hybrids because a few people don't understand Trifield meters." For a copy of his hybrid analysis go to ElectromagneticHealth.org.

Note people who are electrically sensitive often feel better in lower-electronics, older cars in general. In the Prius mentioned above, there were various electronics, including many computers. Hartman says *all* newer cars, not just the hybrids, employ similar electronics, with their ELFs and often higher frequency RF. With respect to higher frequencies "the reality is you probably get more intense RF from outside just driving down the street in an average city."

Self-Protection While Traveling

#36. What should one do to combat the exposure in airplanes?

MH: Some people wear clothing made of RF-reflecting material. RF-reflecting fabric can be found at www.safelivingtechnologies.ca or www.EMFSafetyStore.com.

CR: Airlines clearly need to be educated, however, about the dangers of a plane full of people turning on their cell phones on landing while inside a metal plane. And they need to understand the hazards of allowing in-flight use of wireless and mobile phones, which many airlines are now considering. **This would effectively limit airplane transportation options for many people.**

There are other forms of electromagnetic exposure from airplanes, as well, such as low frequency magnetic fields at 400 Hertz, cosmic radiation, and when landing and taking off, radar.

Before take-off and after landing, if you are sensitive and sitting next to someone who is about to make a call, don't hesitate to explain you are sensitive to EMF. Word needs to get out about the hazards of 2nd hand radiation exposure.

Unfortunately, several airlines are reported to be preparing to test Wi-Fi in flight, including American Airlines, Southwest, Alaska, Virgin America and Jet Blue, according to Macworld, Jul 16, 2008. Ireland's Ryanair is rolling out Wi-Fi for both data and voice. When you travel, inquire as to the availability of Wi-Fi aboard planes and **choose the no-frills airlines not offering it.**

#37. What can I do to protect myself in a wireless hotel room so I don't awaken with brain fog? Are there any hotel chains that you know of not installing wireless in rooms?

MH: Although this is slightly off topic, I travel with a meter and decide which bed I am going to sleep in based on the readings I get. Often the bed closest to the window has higher exposure from antennas outside the hotel. I try to stay in hotels that have wired internet hookup in rooms rather than Wi-Fi. I also carry a microsurge meter and 4 filters to reduce dirty electricity in my hotel room. I did this recently in Houston and felt quite good in my hotel room. The day I was leaving I packed my bags but had some time before going to the airport and worked at the desk in my hotel room and began to feel quite ill. I was sitting near the window and had packed the GS filters and was exposed to both dirty electricity and RF.

CR: Someone needs to educate the hotel industry about the hazards of electromagnetic pollution. Hotels want people to get a good night's sleep, but they clearly have no idea that putting in wireless technology depletes melatonin and impairs sleep, and has neurological effects on the brain. Hard wired connections for internet is what they should be installing instead. I recently visited a Marriott hotel, and it had a hard wired internet connection in the bedroom, fortunately, but I don't know if that's the situation at all Marriott hotels.

I have found in general that the higher end the hotel the more likely it will have wired connections, but one always needs to ask. There are also some hotels with Wi-Fi where it can be turned off. Some people find B&B's a better bet in terms of not having wireless, but call first to find out, and monasteries and retreat centers are another great option and also less expensive. When there are no good hotel options, some people end up staying with friends, or even, in cases of extreme sensitivity, sleep in the car, because they view the trade off in terms of the next day's productivity as too great. It is best to completely avoid sleeping in environments with Wi-Fi, especially when your body needs a good rest.

Recently I visited a charming old hotel, in fact an historic landmark. Levels of microwave radiation ranged from 597-1284 nW/cm^2, extremely high levels. As the saying goes, you can not judge a book by its cover. Measuring, as we continue to stress, is the only way of knowing what level of microwave radiation, or other electromagnetic frequencies, are present.

When you visit hotels ask them to create "Wireless Free Zones", just as many offer "Smoke Free" sections today. Speak up about your concerns on this issue or it will only get more difficult to find a decent night's sleep.

#38. Some people feel worse around Wi-Fi. Is constant Wi-Fi exposure worse than cell phone radiation?

CR: According to Stan Hartman, "One reason Wi-Fi can be more dangerous even than cell phones is because it transmits at full power, rather than having a smart system like a phone does that uses only as much transmitting power as it needs at a given time. Wi-Fi is also often on 24/7, and there is evidence that non-ionizing radiation has a cumulative effect, like non-ionizing radiation (See Question #17, *What Evidence is There For Cumulative Effects of Microwave Radiation?*). Also note that if the computer is not on, but the router still is on, you will be exposed to full power microwave pulses from the router every few seconds, so people should be advised never to turn off the computer while leaving a wireless router on. Both should be turned off together.

#39. Are there dangers in wearing clothing made of shielding fabrics? For example, if I wear a baseball cap made out of shielding material—I can understand it would shield my head from frequencies but what would happen to the frequencies that get into my body from elsewhere—do they get trapped in the brain area, becoming dangerous, because I am wearing the hat?

MH: Wearing shielding inside a hat can reduce your exposure if you are using a cell phone, and wearing RF-reflective fabric can reduce your body exposure, but note in some situations it can also increase exposures, so caution is advised. See Camilla Rees' comments, below.

CR: Some scientists reason that if the microwaves from the phone get under the shielding hat, along with all the other microwave sources from the environment, they will be reflected by it back into the brain. Similarly, if you use a cell phone near a metal door, for instance, you'll get an extra dose of radiation. Shielding in a hat, thus, may indeed reduce the intensity of the direct radiation exposure from the phone, but it could also increase it, and increase overall exposure from the environment *even while not using the phone.*

Humans: Radiofrequency Guidelines & Effects

Power Density (μW/cm^2)

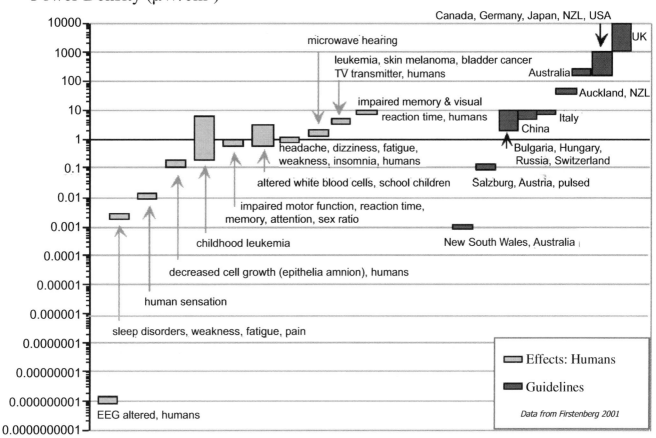

Human Health

Human Health Impacts of EMF/RF

#40. What are the common symptoms of microwave radiation exposure from cell phones, wireless etc?

CR: See Section I - ***"Are You Electrically Sensitive?"*** prepared by Dr. Magda Havas.

Also see ***"Microwave and Radiofrequency Radiation Exposure: A Growing Environmental Health Crisis"*** by Cindy Sage, found on the San Francisco Medical Society's website. It contains a lengthy list of EMF related symptoms and conditions.

These include "changes in cell membrane function, major changes in calcium metabolism and cellular signal communication, cell proliferation, activation of proto-oncogenes, activation of HSP heat shock proteins as if heating has occurred when it has not, and cell death. Resulting effects reported in the scientific literature include DNA breaks and chromosome aberrations, increased free radical production, cell stress and premature aging, changes in brain function including memory loss, learning impairment, headaches and fatigue, sleep disorders, neurodegenerative conditions, reduction in melatonin secretion and cancer."

http://www.sfms.org/AM/Template.cfm?Section=Home&CONTENTID=1770&TEMPLATE=/CM/HTMLDisplay.cfm&SECTION=Article_Archives

Another resource re. symptoms of cell phone radiation is by Santini 2001, La Presse Medicale, http://www.emrnetwork.org/position/santini_english_pm.pdf, which ranks symptoms experienced by distance to the cell phone transmitter. Chart of these symptoms is displayed on page 34.

And finally, another excellent resource can be found at www.waveguide.org/library/studies.html, called EMF/RFR Bioeffects and Public Policy.

#41. Dr. Olle Johansson has said that *everyone* exposed to EMFs registers an inflammatory reaction in the mast cells on the skin, whether or not they feel it. I think everyone is EMF sensitive and just vary in the disease of choice. Would this make sense?

MH: That is why the "illness" is called electro-hyper-sensitivity. We are all electromagnetic and hence sensitive. Those who are "hyper" sensitive respond more severely to lower exposures.

CR: Olle Johansson, Assoc. Professor in Experimental Dermatology, Department of Neuroscience, Karolinska Institute in Sweden, says, "What we have found is that among persons with the functional impairment electrohypersensitivity as well as among normal healthy volunteers you find, in the first group, a highly significant increase in mast cell basal level numbers, and in the second group 2/3 get a similar increase when placed in front of normal household TVs and computer screens. The latter group did not report any subjective sensations, however, they still revealed a classical irradiation damage picture in their skin biopsies. I agree, everyone is EMF sensitive, but only 2-10% (depending on report) reports to have the functional impairment electrohypersensitivity."

#42. I find it terribly wrong the telecom industry has rights to affect my DNA. How much evidence is there that DNA is being impacted, and what are the known consequences of the DNA damage to date?

CR: According to Henry Lai, PhD, author of Chapter 6 of the BioInitiative Report, *"Evidence for Genotoxic Effects"*, of the studies on radiofrequency radiation and DNA damage (28 studies), 50% reported effects; of micronucleus studies (29 studies) 55% reported effects; and of chromosome and genome effects (21 studies) 62% reported effects.

Please note also that both ELF and RF can significantly affect a growing fetus. See the chapter on this in B. Blake Levitt's *"Electromagnetic Fields: A Consumer's Guide to the Issues"*. Levitt says effects can be direct to the fetus through external exposures, through maternal pathways, or through damage to the father's sperm. She says effects can be caused by stress hormones to both the mother and fetus, as well, with the potential amplification of exposures in the conductive amniotic fluid, and through cytokines and inflammatory responses. Levitt also suspects EMF from Doppler ultrasound used routinely in obstetric practice may be harming fetuses, and says autism rates skyrocketed upon its use.

#43. How quickly does a cell phone affect the brain? Is it impacting its structure or function? Are the neurotransmitter levels affected—potentially linking wireless technologies to the depression epidemic?

MH: Change in brainwave activity can be almost immediate although we don't know exactly what the full consequence of this is at present. We have evidence that microwaves increase permeability of the blood brain barrier and hence more rapid movement of substances into and out of the brain, which would affect brain chemistry. There is also evidence that ELF magnetic fields affect melatonin and neurotransmitter levels, although the mechanism by which this happens is not known. We also know serotonin is a precursor for melatonin and serotonin is involved in depression. Most of the anti-depressant drugs are SSRI (selective serotonin-reuptake inhibitors) and are designed for those people with a serotonin deficiency.

CR: Dr. Eric Braverman, MD, author of *The Edge Effect* and expert in the brain's global impact on illness and health says, "There is no question EMFs have a major effect on neurological functioning. They slow our brain waves and affect our long-term mental clarity. We should minimize exposures as much as possible to optimize neurotransmitter levels and prevent deterioration of health".

#44. What are the consequences of the stated increased permeability of the blood-brain barrier?

CR: Anything that does not belong in the brain, that passes from the bloodstream through the blood brain barrier into the brain, presents a potential danger. These might be toxins, like chemicals and metals, or proteins like albumin. Also, bacteria and viruses. The purpose of the barrier is to prevent things from getting into the brain, so EMF/RF increasing its permeability is of very serious concern. The blood-brain barrier helps maintains homeostasis and a constant intracerebral pressure. Damaging this barrier is believed by some scientists to predispose to strokes, as well as to other neurological illnesses such as Parkinson's, MS, ALS, Alzheimer's, autism, etc. According to Deitrich Klinghardt, MD of the Institute for Neurobiology, EMF also affects the gut barrier leading to 'leaky gut' and food and environmental allergies.

#45. How much evidence is there linking EMF/RF to Parkinson's Disease?

MH: We know that radio frequencies in the kHz range affect people with neurological diseases, including multiple sclerosis, but evidence for Parkinson's is still inconclusive. We need more research for Parkinson's Disease and other neurological disorders.

CR: It has been reported that Dr. Albert Giedde of Univ. of Aarhus, Denmark, an authority on both Parkinson's and PET scans, is doing interesting research in this area, as yet unpublished.

#46. With autism now at epidemic levels—has a relationship between autism and ELF/EMF been studied?

MH: We have some anecdotal evidence that autistic children improve if the power quality in their environment is improved.

CR: At present, there is not much scientific evidence for a relationship between ELF/EMF and autism, but there has not been much study. Many leading physicians working with children on the spectrum strongly suspect there is a connection, and research funding is very much needed. At a recent medical conference, Dr. Deitrich Klinghardt, MD, PhD of Kirkland, WA reported he measured EMF body voltage levels in the sleeping locations of mothers of autistic children, and measured the same for mothers of healthy children. He found the average body voltage levels in the sleeping locations of mothers who had healthy children to be 224 mV (range 12-480) vs. 1872 mV (range 380-6040) for the mothers of autistic children (with anything above 80 millivolts considered very bad). He also measured the body voltage in the childrens' bed locations, and found, on average, levels of 120 mV (range 0-230) in the healthy children vs. 1082 mV (range 420-4900) in the autistic children. Dr. Klinghardt also measured microwave power density in the sleeping location of the mothers and found on average a level of 290 mW/sq. meter (range 110-1710) in the mothers sleeping location where the child was neurologically impaired versus 14 mW/sq. meter (range 0-67) in the sleeping locations of the mothers who gave birth to healthy children. Given some estimates are that approximately 1 in 50 children are born with autism today, up from 1 in 150 in 2002, the EMF connection with autism must be aggressively studied.

#47. Do EMF exposures worsen reaction to toxic chemicals, mold and other allergens?

CR: There is disagreement on this topic, with some scientists believing much more study is needed, and others who say the meta-analysis by Juutilainen et al (2006) offers proof. I would recommend consulting experts in the area of chemical sensitivity at the Environmental Health Center in Dallas, TX. There are many studies on EMF and chemical carcinogens of which they would likely be aware. Some studies show EMF exposure makes the chemical damage worse, including RF increasing the toxicity of formaldehyde and carbon monoxide (Shandala MG and Vinogradov GI. Immunological Effects of Microwave Action. *Gigiyena i Sanitariya* 10:34-38, 1978. JPRS 72956, pp. 1621). An article with additional references on this subject, *Microwaves Imitate Pesticides* by Lucinda Grant, can be found at http://www.emrnetwork.org/sensitivity/mwimitate.pdf.

Also of note, a report published recently in Electromagnetic Biology and Medicine, *"Increased Concentrations of Certain Persistent Organic Pollutants in Subjects with Self-Reported Electromagnetic Hypersensitivity—A Pilot Study"*, by Lennart Hardell et al, shows the concentration of certain persistent organic pollutants (POPs) in people with electrohypersensitivity is higher than in controls. Further investigation of the connection between body burden of chemicals and electro-hypersensitivity must be explored. (*Electromagnetic Biology and Medicine*, 27:197-203, 2008)

#48. Can RF and power transmission radiation reverse cancer remission? (Question from a patient who was in remission and sent home to a house with power lines over the property—cancer came back very shortly afterwards)

MH: Some anecdotal evidence suggests that patients who have cancer remission are more likely to have the cancer return if they go back to live or work in an electromagnetically dirty environment. There is also evidence that tamoxifen, which is used for estrogen positive breast cancer, is less effective when the magnetic field exposure is above 12 milligauss.

#49. Is it possible to isolate the symptoms and health effects of electromagnetic energy, when we are also being exposed daily to toxins such as pesticides, percholate in water, hormones in foods, etc?

MH: Yes. We have done studies in U.S. schools where the only thing that was changed was the dirty electricity. So we can associate some improvements in health directly to power quality.

#50. Is there a connection between EMF/RF exposure and low thyroid function?

MH: We have some evidence for RF exposure but I am unfamiliar with evidence for thyroid dysfunction and ELF EMF exposure. There are numerous studies dating back to the 1970s indicating microwaves influence the thyroid.

CR: In research done by medical epidemiologist Sam Milham, MD at the La Quinta Middle School in La Quinta, CA, which had high levels of dirty power, there was a 13-fold excess in thyroid cancer above what would otherwise be expected. (See *A New Electromagnetic Exposure Metric: High Frequency Voltage Transients Associated With Increased Cancer Incidence in Teachers in a California School*", published in the American Journal of Industrial Medicine.) (http://www.ncbi.nlm.nih.gov/pubmed/18512243)

One study on RF effects on thyroid hormones was published in Toxicology Letter (2005 Jul 4; 157(3):257-62. Epub 2005 April 11). The study showed that 900MHz EMF emitted by cellular telephones decrease serum TSH and T3-T4 levels.

#51. Is there a connection between exponential growth in EMF/RF exposures and the obesity epidemic?

MH: I am unaware of any research in this area.

CR: It seems common sense that research dollars should be allocated to explore this given the sharp rise in obesity over the past 15 years, including in pets, just as the wireless industry has expanded exponentially.

#52. Can you speak to the actual physiological disruption that occurs with exposure—ex: calcium ion mobilization?

MH: Physiological disruption with exposure to RFR and/or ELF include increased permeability of the blood-brain barrier, increased activity of the enzyme ODC, which is associated with cancers, increased calcium flux, reduced melatonin (in some studies), increase in stress protein production, changes in blood sugar, DNA breaks, altered cell proliferation, altered blood pressure and heart rate, dermatological effects, cognitive dysfunction, etc.

CR: The scientists who prepared the BioInitiative Report reviewed over 2,000 research studies, and synthesized the current state of our understanding of physiological processes from ELF and RF (www.BioInitiative.org).

Another review of the science worth reading is the *"Analysis of Health and Environmental Effects of Proposed San Francisco Earthlink Wi-Fi Network"* prepared by Dr. Magda Havas, found at http://www.energyfields.org/pdfs/WiF-SNAFU-Havas-Science.pdf

#53. Is there a connection between the rise in insulin resistance and EMF exposure?

MH: Possibly. One study in Switzerland (Altpeter et al. 1995) showed an increase in the incidence of diabetics with proximity to a short-wave transmitter. Diabetic subjects experimentally exposed to 60-Hz magnetic fields had higher blood glucose levels above 0.6 microT (6 mG) (Litovitz et al. 1994). In vitro studies show that insulin release is reduced when Islets of Langerhans are exposed to magnetic fields (Sakurai et al 2004). This would result in high blood sugar levels. The authors of this study conclude: "it might be desirable for diabetic patients who have insufficient insulin secretion from pancreatic islets to avoid exposure to ELF MF". There is also evidence that stress (physical or psychological) increases blood glucose levels in diabetics and that exposure to EMF stimulates production of stress proteins in laboratory animals (Blank and Goodman 2004).

#54. Is electrical hypersensitivity recognized as a disability?

MH: Yes, in Sweden, and recently in Canada.

CR: In the US it is recognized by the US Access Board, but this does not get electrohypersensitive individuals any help in practice because no official action has been taken. Much more needs to be done to accommodate those who are suffering and who no longer have the full access to society they once did. A suit claiming violation of the Americans With Disabilities Act is under consideration. **Please sign EMF Petition to Congress at www.ElectromagneticHealth.org.**

How to Keep the Body Functioning Optimally in High EMF/RF Environments

#55. Are there any vitamins or natural substances that one can take to reduce EMF sensitivity? (Especially if one already suffers from occasional tremors due to electrical sensitivity)

MH:
1. <u>Reduce your exposure.</u>

2. <u>Improve your immune system</u> with vitamins, minerals, nutritious food, exercise, and other non-pharmaceutical supplements.

3. <u>Reduce your toxic load</u> safely and slowly with antioxidants, colonics, removal of mercury fillings, etc. Do this under the guidance of a qualified medical practitioner who understands proper detoxification methods and has experience working with EHS.

CR: Some physicians have found it is often the case that sensitive people have excess amounts of heavy metals, mercury amalgam fillings and/or hidden infections. Low (and sometimes high) mineral status is also common. There is no one-size-fits-all protocol. Care must be individualized. Gunnar Heuser, MD of UCLA recommends melatonin levels be assessed. Other physicians, such as Eric Braverman, MD in New York, author of *The Edge Effect*, say neurotransmitter levels are affected by EMFs, and that they can be supported with individualized supplement/diet/drug protocols as described in this book. Lisa Nagy, MD of the Preventive and Environmental Health Alliance says potassium and calcium help some patients with electrical sensitivity, and that mixed dental metals leading to oral galvanism should be assessed as a means to potentially reducing symptoms in some people.

Dr. Deitrich Klinghardt in Kirkland, WA gives a course on EMF for physicians with an added focus on assessing and remediating the physical environment (www.neuraltherapy.com). He reviews how: 1) body weight, body-mass index, bonedensity, etc. alter the conductivity and receptivity of the organism, 2) water and electrolyte levels alter the antenna function of the organism (dehydration being protective), 3) touching the earth discharges static electricity, 4) heavy metals in the brain act as microantennae (Y. Omura), concentrate EMF-radiation into the brain and increase reception, 5) dental amalgams increase reception of radiowaves, microcurrent from cell phone broadcasting and from all ambient fields, 6) genes regulate the metal detoxifying enzymes and can predetermine people to be electro-sensitive, 7) loss of myelin (i.e. insulation) increases reception (MS, Lyme, auto immune processes, etc.), and finally 8) there is a synergistic effect from geopathic earth radiation, metallic objects in the home, electric and magnetic field appliances and household current and incoming microwave from cell phones. Klinghardt stresses the importance of regular detoxification efforts to unburden the body of neurotoxins generated by microorganisms in response to EMFs.

According to Leo Galland, MD of the Foundation for Integrated Medicine in New York City, one of New York's leading internists, people with EMF sensitivity very often have food, mold and chemical sensitivities. "I recommend for my EMF sensitive patients that they eat organic food, avoid sweets and foods high in yeast or mold (bread, dried fruits, fruit juices, vinegar, alcohol), and be tested for food allergies. An anti-inflammatory diet, high in vegetables, sources of omega-3 fats like organic flax seed and wild salmon, and herbs and spices like turmeric and ginger, can also be helpful." Dr. Galland's anti-inflammatory program is called The Fat Resistance Diet (www.fatresistancediet.com).

Finally, there is an excellent article, *Living With Hypersensitivity, A Survival Guide*, on the WEEP Initiative website, a Canadian EMF resource site. http://weepinitiative.org/livingwithEHS.

#56. What can I do to optimize neurological functioning given the daily assaults from these technologies? Are there any proactive steps one can take?

CR: See Section III, *"Electromagnetic (EMF) Safety Recommendations"* as well as question #55, above. Also see *"Reducing Electromagnetic Frequency Exposure May Improve Your Health"* on http://www.naturalnews.com/022926.html

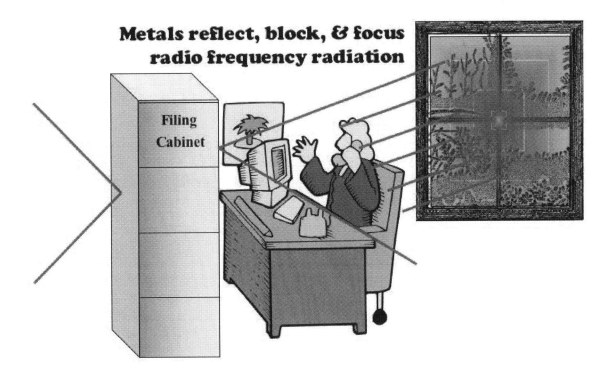

Metals reflect, block, & focus radio frequency radiation

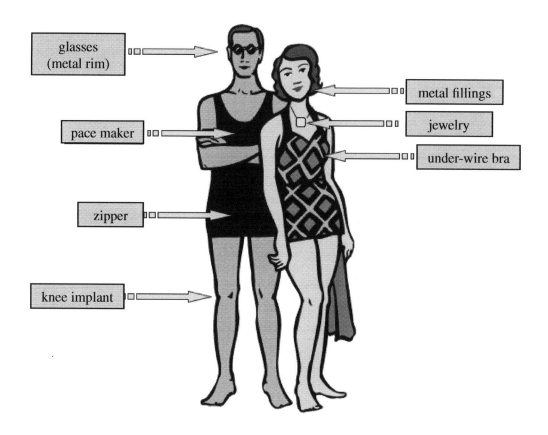

EMF Impact on Drug Absorption

#57. I heard EMF is affecting the efficacy of the breast cancer drug Tamoxifen. Does this suggest it is affecting the efficacy of other pharmaceutical drugs as well?

MH: The evidence we have for tamoxifen comes from *in vitro* studies with human breast cancer cells and shows that there is a slight but statistically significant decrease in tamoxifen's effectiveness in reducing the growth of estrogen-responsive breast cancer cells when exposed to 12 milligauss magnetic fields. There is, as yet, no evidence in human subjects for tamoxifen. For some pharmaceutical drugs, it is unadvised for people to be exposed to sunlight (which is part of the electromagnetic spectrum) so this interaction with EM frequencies and drugs is well known for light but less well known for other frequencies.

CR: Microwave radiation has been shown to increase the effects of morphine, interfere with Librium (sedative, central nervous system depressant); increase the effects of Haldol (antipsychotic, for nervous, mental and emotional conditions); and counteract the effects of amphetamines (central nervous system stimulants). It also increased the toxicity of Cardiazole, a drug taken off the market by the FDA in 1982.

(See *On the Nature of Electromagnetic Field Interactions with Biological Systems,* AH Frey, ed., RG Landes Co., Austin, 1994, pp. 9-28; Also, Lai H, Horita A, Chou CK, Guy AW. Psychoactive-Drug Response is Affected by Acute Low-Level Microwave Irradiation. *Bioelectromagnetics* 1983;4(3):205-14; and Baranski S and Czerski P. *Biological Effects of Microwaves.* Dowden, Hutchinson & Ross, Stroudsburg, 1976.)

Health Industry Use of EMF/RF:

#58. What about exposure from X-rays—mammograms, dental x-rays etc?

MH: X-rays produce ionizing radiation that is known to be harmful. That is why we now have such stringent guidelines on X-ray exposure for both patients and technicians and that is why you wear a lead apron around your body when your teeth are being X-rayed.

CR: At this panel we are focused on microwave radiation, which is part of the non-ionizing radiation portion of the electromagnetic spectrum. The ionizing portion of the electromagnetic spectrum comprises ultraviolet radiation, x-rays, gamma rays, beta rays, alpha particles and cosmic rays, and the non-ionizing portion comprises infrared radiation, microwaves, radio waves and Extremely Low Frequency (ELF). As people commonly understand, there are serious negative health effects from X-rays, as they can strip electrons from the atom. Much less understood among the general public, health professionals and scientists are the health effects from lower power microwave radiation we are discussing here. The heating effect is unquestioned, but the non-thermal effects are not well understood and are politically contentious. It is important the public health community get up to speed on this issue as there is research showing non-ionizing radiation may be a universal carcinogen like ionizing radiation.

#59. Is it true frequencies are now being used in research to treat cancer?

MH: Yes and they are also used to heal bone fractures and for soft-tissue healing.

CR: Excellent article on this in *Physics Today,* August 2007 (http://ptonline.aip.org/getpdf/servlet/GetPDFServlet?filetype=pdf&id=PHTOAD000060000008000019000001&idtype=cvips).

#60. Are hospital environments safe for patients from an EMF perspective?

CR: In addition to X-rays, MRI, CT Scans, etc, wireless technology is used extensively in hospital environments. Radio frequency identification tags (RFID) are now used for medical equipment inventory management and theft prevention, and wireless patient monitoring is the norm, both requiring hospital-wide antennas and receivers. In addition, the staff in many hospitals wear wireless monitors today so their whereabouts can be known at all times.

In a recent study, *"Electromagnetic Interference From Radio Frequency Identification Inducing Potentially Hazardous Incidents in Critical Care Medical Equipment"* (Remko van der Togt; Erik Jan van Lieshout; Reinout Hensbroek; E. Beinat; J. M. Binnekade; P. J. M. Bakker JAMA. 2008;299(24):2884-2890), it was shown wireless communications cause errors in critical care equipment 30% of the time, 20% of the time considered hazardous. Examples cited were wireless communications 1) turning breathing machines off, 2) making mechanical syringe pumps delivering medications stop delivering medication, and 3) causing external pacemakers to malfunction.

Additionally, there is serious concern about the telecom companies starting to use the 'white spaces' on the spectrum between TV channels, which has been known to disable heart monitoring equipment, and other equipment, in hospitals. (http://news.cnet.com/8301-10784_3-9930441-7.html).

There was a post recently from a Parkinson's patient on a list serve of the Collaborative for Health and the Environment's EMF Working Group. A patient had visited the Emergency Room where her "deep brain stimulation system" was turned off by a wireless scanner that was scanning an RFID tag on the pain medication she was being given. Within minutes of exposure to the wireless scanner her Parkinson's motor symptoms reappeared.

Outside of hospitals, similar situations unfortunately routinely occur in wireless environments for patients using critical care equipment, such as pacemakers and defibrillators, which are set off by wireless security systems, wireless theft detection systems and other electronic devices.

In the Operating Room, there are even 'smart' surgical sponges today, detectable with a microwave wand, to make sure surgeons do not leave sponges inside patients. In a cardiac patients room at a local hospital in Boulder, CO, RF levels measured 3.4 microwatts per square centimeter, an extraordinarily high level of exposure, and levels of dirty electricity were off the scale. This would not be a room one would want to recover in post-surgery for long, especially if one is electrically sensitive.

So, from an EMF perspective, hospitals may not be safe environments for electrically sensitive people, or for people who use electrically sensitive devices. In both cases we are talking about electromagnetic interference, whether within a body or in equipment.

Environmental Health

EMF Impact on Animals & Nature

#61. Have any of you done research on the effect of microwave radiation on bees?

CR: CR: See recent article on this:
http://www.hese-project.org/hese-uk/en/niemr/kompetenz_beekeepers.pdf

There is also a new booklet out, in German only at the moment, that is reported to be excellent: *"Bees, Birds and Humans: The Destruction of Nature by Electrosmog"* by Ulrich Warnke, 2008. (German name "Bienen, Völker und Menschen") Contact: bienenbroschuere@kompetenzinitiative.de

#62. Is it true that birds are dropping out of the sky by the millions due to EMF? Are environmental organizations on to this issue yet?

MH: Most of the bird deaths, to my knowledge, are due to birds colliding with large towers, particularly those with flashing lights. RF energy also affects bird behavior and breeding success and may interfere with migration patterns.

CR: According to B. Blake Levitt, author of *"Electromagnetic Fields, A Consumer's Guide to the Issues and How to Protect Ourselves,"* and Editor of "Cell Towers, Wireless Convenience? Or Environmental Hazard?" radiofrequency radiation (RF) is a form of energetic air pollution capable of affecting a myriad of species, not just humans. She says, "One tower at 150 feet is thought to account for as many as 3,000 songbird deaths a month in some migratory flyways. Multiply that by the number of towers already present and those being built daily and the figure of likely bird deaths attributable to this technology does get into the millions." Levitt says according to Albert M. Manville, II, Ph.D., head of the Division of Migratory Bird Management at the U.S. Fish and Wildlife Service a conservative estimate of bird deaths attributable to towers would be around 3-to-5 million a year.

She adds, "It has been known for years that the songbird population of North America is plummeting. Only recently were towers considered a factor. But the big question remains: Is the problem solely one of tower construction acting as obstacles in migratory pathways? Or could something else be involved? What if RF is acting as an attractant to birds? Avian eye and beak areas are known to be loaded with a magnetic material called magnetite. In a recent paper, noted American ornithologist Robert Beason and Peter Semm of Germany found that a pulsed RF signal (at 900 MHz, modulated at 217 Hz) similar to that of mobile phone technology, resulted in changes in neural activity in more than half of the avian brain cells being tested. Seventy-six percent increased their rates of neuronal firing by an average of 3.5 fold."

Levitt goes on to say, "Recent research in Europe found that sparrows and other birds abandoned areas with increased RF backgrounds from cell towers. Other species affected included bats, invertebrates, insects, domestic animals, trees and some bushes." She says, "Another study found increased rates of infertility and growth abnormalities in test animals at some distance from 'antenna parks' where exposure levels were well below standards. By the fifth generation, test animals were permanently infertile. And several studies of cows near radio towers found agitation, lower milk production and birth defects in calves."

Levitt, a long time science writer, former New York Times writer and passionate environmentalist emphasizes, "Something is clearly going on here". She says, "Some environmental organizations, like the Berkshire-Litchfield Environmental Council, the Forest Conservancy Council, and Friends of the Earth have taken an interest in the broader impacts of this technology on wildlife. The Natural Resources Defense Council has taken on the issue of the military's use of sonar and its effects on marine wildlife but they have not gotten their teeth into ambient non-ionizing radiation beyond that."

I learned recently, in an encouraging move, in February 2008, a federal court of appeals issued a ruling ordering the FCC to evaluate the potential adverse effects of communications towers on migratory bird populations of the Gulf Coast. http://pacer.cadc.uscourts.gov/docs/common/opinions/200802/06-1165a.pdf

The court criticized the FCC for refusing to consult with the U.S. Fish & Wildlife Service when approving such towers and also for failing to sufficiently involve the public in its tower approval process. It said, "The Commission provides public notice to individual tower applications only after approving them". The FCC was found to violate federal law by approving towers in this way with no environmental review. Public interest law firm Earthjustice brought the case against the FCC and the CTIA (cellular industry association) on behalf of the American Bird Conservancy and the Forest Conservation Council. To support non-profit law firm Earthjustice's commendable work for this and other environmental causes, go to: http://www.earthjustice.org/about_us/index.html

There is no question the environmental movement as a whole is way behind the curve and needs to get involved and make this their issue, too. It is essential groups in this area begin to develop more of a focus on human health, instead of focusing mostly in *energy efficiency*. Attention should be paid to microwave radiation from cell phones, wireless hazards and the serious health concerns regarding compact fluorescent bulbs, Broadband Over Power line technology employed in SmartGrids, dirty electricity generated by solar panels and the coming Wi-Max, to blanket us all shortly.

Measuring Exposures & Exposure Standards

Measuring EMF/RF

#63. Are there tools to measure the amount of EMFs or microwaves in our environment?

MH: Yes. Different tools measure different things. There are many brands and models and it can be confusing for the layperson if one is not familiar with the science of measurement. Here are 3 meters I recommend for the basics:

ELF EMF (extremely low frequency electric and magnetic fields): Trifield meter less than $200. This meter is easy to use and relatively inexpensive. It has an omni directional antenna, which means it doesn't matter how you hold it and it will give the same reading.

It does have some shortcomings however, as do all meters, and it has to be used with some understanding of what someone is measuring and what other frequencies are present in the environment. For example, in a low frequency environment the magnetic field reading should be reliable but if radio frequencies are present it will give abnormally high readings. One can ask for a "flat frequency" Trifield meter that provides more reliable readings in a high RF environment. The electric field is normally difficult to measure as the human body influences the reading and this is true for the trifield meter as well. The RF/MW part of the Trifield meter is virtually useless for any type of monitoring.

RF (radio frequency/microwave): An inexpensive meter ($200) that is sensitive (32 nW/cm^2) and accurate (+/-2.4 dB) is the Electrosmog Meter available at www.EMFSafetyStore.com (Cat. #WAH492). It has a frequency range of 50 MHz to 3.5 GHz, is ideal for digital or analog RF signals, has an omni- and uni-directional antenna and many other options. It is probably the best meter at a low price. A wider spectrum and more expensive 8GHz version has just been introduced as well.

DE (dirty electricity): Microsurge meter $135 plus one GS filter $39.

CR: Of the inexpensive combination magnetic/electric meters, Hartman's favorite is the Gigahertz Solutions ME3030B ("Digital Combination Meter"). It has a few drawbacks in functionality, being slow and having a too-low-frequency sensitivity so you have to hold it very steady, but the readings are accurate and it also has an audio output. For the nontechnical layperson, he likes a simple and inexpensive magnetic field finder called the budget Buzz Stick. Another one he especially likes, a bit higher price, is the FW Bell 4080, which is omnidirectional, has +/- 2% accuracy and a broad frequency band from 25Hz to 1,000 kHz.

Hartman cautions that laypeople should not be attempting to measure RF fields, unless they want to spend a lot of money on a professional, high end accurate meter and then take the time to learn how to use it. For finding (vs. measuring) RF/MW, he likes the Zapchecker 185 http://zapchecker.com/zc185.html. The Zapchecker, he says, is very broadband, between 3 MHz and 5 GHz (though actually useful up to 6 GHz or higher), distinguishes between digital and analog signals, and is less than $200. "It has an analog display and is fast", he says, "which is an essential feature when trying to detect RF/MW. Many much more expensive meters will miss quick pulses entirely because they have to take the time to try to measure them accurately, which can take as much as 2 seconds".

For a review of worthwhile RF, magnetic and electric field meters, please go to www.EMFSafetyStore.com.

#64. What are people called who have these skills? Would an electrician be equipped to assess the EMF/RF environment?

MH: Most electricians are unaware of the research in this area. We need more people who are qualified to do measurements and remediation properly.

CR: One strategy would be to source a qualified professional and have that person work with your local electrician. Sources of experts might be the Institute of Bau Biology & Ecology, the Electromagnetic Field Testing Association or eventually, once they update their education to thoroughly address EMF issues, LEED (Leadership in Energy & Environmental Design) environmental consultants certified by the U.S. Green Building Council.

Other measurement resources include Larry Gust (www.gustenvironmental.com), Peter Sierck (www.etandt.com) and Stephen Scott (www.EMFServices.com) in California; Stan Hartman in Colorado (www.radsafe.net); Vicky Warren in Tennessee (www.wehliving. org); Will Spates in Florida (www.ietbuildinghealth.com); Sal LaDuca in New Jersey (http://www.emfrelief.com); Dave Stetzer in Wisconsin (www.stetzerelectric.com); Jim Beal in TX (www.emfinterface.com) and Dan Stih in New Mexico (www.healthylivingspaces.com). In Ontario, Canada, there is Kevin Byrne (www.dirtyelectricity.ca), Robert Steller (www. breathing-easy.net) and Rob Metzinger (www.safelivingtechnologies.ca).

#65. Are there reliable meters for measuring RFR?

CR: Yes. See Section V, "Books, Videos, Journals & Websites, etc.", for sources of measuring equipment, including: Less EMF, Safe Living Technologies, EMFSafetyStore, Alpha Labs and the Microwave News websites. However, please note the advice given earlier that laypeople might consider a meter that *finds* as opposed to *measures* RF, as there is a steep learning curve involved particularly for RF measurement equipment.

Exposure Standards & Issues

#66. Is it true that Austria and Russia have far more protective standards? Is this what the US should emulate?

MH: Guidelines vary around the world. Guidelines differ by 5 orders of magnitude for RFR, 3 orders of magnitude for ELF magnetic fields, and 2 orders of magnitude for ELF electric fields.

CR: Some say Russia's lower limits are not adequate to provide any real protection, and also note Salzburg, Austria's voluntary standards for certain antennas are not enforced. Liechtenstein, in November of 2008, became the first country to mandate 10x lower emission standards to go into effect in 2013. These limits will be in line with the recommendations of the BioInitiative Report. (See http://videos.next-up.org/SfTv/Liechtenstein/AdoptsTheStandardOf06VmBioInitiative/09112008.html)

The U.S. needs to find the conviction and commitment to establish biologically based exposure standards. Concerns about the health impact of microwave and radiofrequency radiation, and about the inadequate exposure standards now used, must be heard by our government leaders. Please sign the **Petition to Congress** at www.ElectromagneticHealth.org.

#67. We are currently revising the code for antennas in Richmond, CA. We are asking for a buffer of 1,000 feet from the new higher powered antennas. Can you advise on a reasonable buffer zone for schools/homes?

MH: What few studies are available show adverse health effects within 400 meters (1200 feet) for cell phone antennas and within 2 km for broadcast antennas. However, it will also depend on your direction from the main beam of the various antennas, number of antennas, power of antennas, amount of metal in your home exposed to these antennas, etc. See comments below.

CR: See Question #30, "How far away do cell phone towers have to be from your home to be 100% safe?" for additional discussion on this topic.

Understand that people who are electrically sensitive can feel effects from some cell towers 2-3 miles away. It is important people take into consideration the power of the antenna(s) and realize 'distance' is not always a useful measure of safety. Also note one can be close to an antenna as the crow flies, but with a mountain in between, so you wouldn't be affected at all. So it is hard to generalize. One must take actual measurements. Also recognize that the power levels coming from antennas on a nearby cell tower could be increased without your knowledge, so it's worthwhile to recheck exposure levels periodically.

Stan Hartman, an environmental consultant experienced in measuring electromagnetic fields, adds,

"It's difficult to generalize about safe distances from cell towers. Putting aside the variables that have to do with personal health, personal genetic profile and so forth, there are also landscape factors to consider – weather, humidity, how many obstructions are between the tower and the subject, what their geometry is, what they're composed of. Then there are the questions of how many antennas are on the tower; their geometry, angle, and beam pattern; the level of cell traffic the tower is serving, how far away the traffic is, the angle of the antennas, etc.

It's very difficult to accurately measure exposure levels in an urban or suburban environment at any distance more than a few hundred yards, because of the profusion of sources and reflections. Even with a directional antenna, you don't know if you're picking up a primary signal or a reflection. There really isn't any way to generalize and answer the question just in terms of distance."

Real Estate Related

Real Estate Valuation Impact

#68. How do you know where the antennas are in your neighborhood? Will close proximity to towers devalue property?

MH: www.antennasearch.com. Type in your address to find out where towers are within 8 miles of your home.

CR: Yes, towers with antennas nearby will impact decision making of savvy buyers. One member of the audience this evening has lost all equity in her home because word got out the radiofrequency radiation was making her family sick, and no one will buy the house.

Communities that have gone 'wireless' will eventually drive people away as residents experience and learn about the health hazards with time.

Apartment living is increasingly difficult for people who are electrically sensitive because of the RF coming from neighbors, not to mention large apartment buildings who take revenue from the cell phone industry in the form of several thousand dollars a month in exchange for agreeing to house telecom antennas on their roofs or internal premises (about which tenants generally have no idea). For these reasons, homes with land around them, if they can be afforded, I believe will become increasingly in demand as more and more people become electrically sensitive.

Be cautious around churches and schools, which sadly often lease their steeples, roofs and property to the wireless industry. One school district in Canada receives $1.3mm in revenue annually leasing space on their property for antennas.

People should inquire where the Sprint/Clearwire/Time Warner/Google Wi-Max antenna system will be installed in their neighborhoods. Property near these high power antennas will be undesirable.

Another antenna-locating resource to know about is www.AntennaWeb.org provided by the Consumer Electronics Broadcasters Association (CEA) and the National Association of Broadcasters (NAB). It identifies, based on *signal strengths*, the location of the best antenna for use with a home satellite system, high-definition television (HDTV) or a traditional analog set.

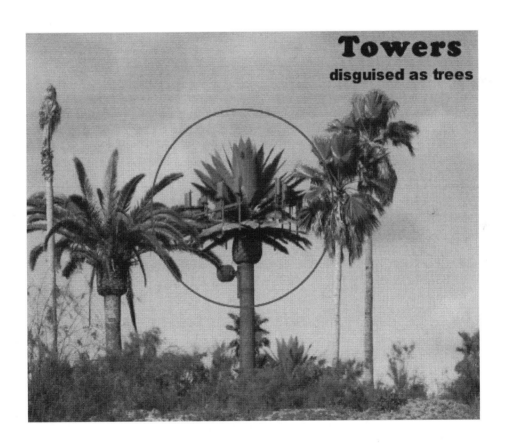

Towers disguised as trees

Public's Right to Know Whereabouts of Towers/Antennas

#69. Is there anything being done to identify to the public the buildings with cell phone towers on the premises?

MH: You can get information about antenna locations that is moderately accurate from www.antennasearch.com. It requires a street address.

CR: It is very instructive to walk around urban areas with an RF meter or audio RF detector!

#70. Also, what is the law regarding access to roofs with towers? (Question was from a telecom installer)

MH: If you get close enough to an antenna you will enter the "near field", which is much more dangerous than the far field. Signage and fencing is required to prevent the public from doing this accidentally.

#71. As a potential renter, or a purchaser of residential property, is disclosure required if there is cell phone equipment in or on or near the building? If not, what are the necessary steps to make this a requirement?

CR: Some states require disclosure of environmental factors that should in theory impact valuation. However, in practice I do not know how well this is enforced, and EMF/RF is probably barely on the radar screen of real estate agents, or renters and buyers at this point.

In fact, large apartment towers will commonly rent space on or in the building for antennas, and in my personal experience no mention is made to tenants whatsoever, even when asked if there are environmental concerns. Find out if there is a cell company antenna on your building at www.antennasearch.com or simply bring someone in to measure RF fields.

From my personal experience measuring RF in many San Francisco neighborhoods, I found street intersections to have a higher prevalence of radiofrequency, making these intersections less desirable to those who want or need to avoid EMF/RF.

Realize sometimes the antennas are visible, and other times they are intentionally concealed within or on a structure, or in church towers or disguised as a tree or behind a façade, etc. It is my opinion that full disclosure to all neighbors should be required in these circumstances.

Another key issue related to real estate that needs addressing is *tenants rights regarding second hand radiation*—from routers, cordless phones, antennas, etc. from neighbors.

People's lives are being devastated by radiofrequency coming from their neighbors, and most people don't even know that their neighbor's RF could be a factor.

Neighborhood Health Surveys

#72. I live within 300 feet from a cell tower and want to conduct an epidemiological survey of my neighborhood. Are there any resources to help me with this?

MH: Contact Janet Newton at www.emrpolicy.org. A survey was designed to give you a sense of how it is affecting people. If you decide to use this survey it is asked that you share the results with EMR Policy Institute for their data bank.

If you are not an epidemiologist, we recommend you work with one to ensure proper method and reliability of the responses, and proper analysis of the data. It is not recommended you administer the survey on your own. Without guidance you could easily jeopardize the validity of the results.

CR: A sample of the Green Audit survey mentioned above is attached herein for your convenience in Section VI, Community Health Survey, and is also printable from www.ElectromagneticHealth.org. Please note a large population would be required to attain statistically significant results.

When a community in the UK decided to do community health assessments pre- and post-cell phone tower erection, however, the provider changed its mind and did not erect the tower.

Note also that the value of a survey such as this is muddied by the tremendous amount of exposure already occurring within peoples homes themselves, and also that the FCC has made it illegal to consider health and environmental effects when siting cell powers. (See Question #104, "What are roles of the EPA, FDA, FCC and other Federal Government Agencies with Respect to Protecting Health from the Health Effects of Radiofrequency Radiation? In Other Words, Who is Protecting Us?"). Thus, it may not help much legally to have conducted a survey, unfortunately, but it still makes worthwhile news, which in and of itself could move the issue forward.

That being said, we highly encourage you to conduct health surveys in your communities before and after the roll out across the nation of high-powered Wi-Max. **NOW IS THE TIME TO CONDUCT A SURVEY** since plans by Sprint, Clearwire, Time Warner Cable and Google are for a very rapid Wi-Max roll-out. It has been reported that half the country is intended to be blanketed in Wi-Max by 2010, and the rest of the country shortly thereafter.

Science and Research Related

Research Issues

#73. Why are all current studies of brain tumors from cell phone use funded by the cell phone industry?

MH: Because the government is NOT funding any studies on RF. Industry has not funded any cell phone studies recently. The latest one I am familiar with came out in 2004.

See article by Henry Lai (2005): "Radiation Danger from Cell Phones? Largest "Experiment" in the World is Under Way". The Trend. University of Washington, College of Engineering. Lai says there have been about 200 studies on the biological effects of cell-phone-related radiation. "When you look at the non-industry sponsored research, about three out of every four papers shows an effect," Lai says.

Then, if you look at the industry-funded research, it's almost the opposite—only one out of every four papers shows an effect." The problem, he adds, is that there is no funding available in the United States that isn't attached to the industry. Lai, for one, refuses to take any more industry money.

http://64.233.167.104/search?q=cache:wgPys0iyjkAJ:www.engr.washington.edu/news/trendsummer05.pdf+Lai+%2B%22industry+funded+research%22+%2B%22cell+phone%22 &hl=en&ct=clnk&cd=3&gl=ca&client=firefox-a

#74. Has the US government taken any interest in the BioInitiative Report?

CR: I would guess most people in the US government have not read or heard of the BioInitiative Report. It has not been covered well by the US media. It is hoped money can be found to further publicize this important review of the ELF/RF research, highlighting the findings of ELF/RF links with specific illnesses. This way, disease-specific associations can see reasons for becoming involved with this issue, and further research funding will naturally follow. If you would like to support publicity on EMF/RF and health, please contact Info@ ElectromagneticHealth.org. There are many funding opportunities available for awareness-raising, education and research on this topic , some of which are outlined in Section VIII - Can You Support Further EMF Advocacy & Research?

Interphone Study

#75. What exactly is the Interphone Study and is it true the results have been delayed for years?

MH: The Interphone study is a multi-nation study originally intended to put health concerns about cell phone use to rest by conducting a very detailed study with large numbers of participants across the globe, thereby increasing the statistical validity of the results. Data from several countries is still forthcoming. Some countries have released the data prematurely because of the long delay in reporting by other countries, and thus in the final report.

CR: According to Louis Slesin, PhD, Editor & Publisher of *Microwave News*, an industry expert who has been tracking developments in this field for decades, "The delay in the release of the Interphone study begs the question: Who speaks for public health? Results from some of the 13 countries participating in Interphone, now published in peer-reviewed journals, point to a long-term tumor risk among heavy users of cell phones. But few of the team members are willing to make public statements about the implications of these findings until the final results of the project are published. At this writing (in the early summer of 2008), drafts of the final paper have been circulating for close to three years! Clearly, there are divisions within the study team, which is stymieing a consensus view of the risks. Meanwhile, the telecoms are marketing mobile phones to younger and younger children. Many of the participating epidemiologists have lost sight of the true mission: *To advise the public of potential health risks and to encourage those who are concerned to take precautionary action.*"

An analysis of the Interphone studies published to date, conducted by L. Lloyd Morgan, BS, presented in June 2008 to the Bioelectromagnetics Society, shows the Interphone Protocol has *serious design flaws that result in significant underestimation of the risk of brain tumors.* These flaws range from selection bias, where controls who agree to participate are more frequent cell phone users than non-participating controls; considering tumors *outside* of the radiation plume as 'exposed'; cell phone use (latency) time, which is too short to expect a tumor diagnosis; defining 'regular user' as persons who use a phone at least 1x a week for six months or more, an unrealistic definition of a 'regular' user; excluding young adults and children (known to be at the greatest risk from exposure to carcinogens); only considering a few brain tumor types, and not others; and excluding brain tumor cases because of death, which of course makes no sense whatsoever. The result of these flaws is that the Interphone studies published to date actually find use of a cellphone protects the users from brain tumors! According to Lloyd Morgan, BS, the *cellphone industry-funded* 13-country Interphone study thus "is not the definitive study it purports to be", as the design flaws have distorted results beyond reason. The only independent cell phone study, a Swedish team led by Dr. Lennart Hardell, has found a consistent risk of brain tumors from cell phone use.

For a copy of Lloyd Morgan's Interphone Study analysis, presented at the Bioelectromagnetics Society, please go to **Media Story Leads** at **www.ElectromagneticHealth.org** where it can be downloaded.

Sources of Dirty Electricity

- computers
- variable speed motors
- television sets
- entertainment units
- energy efficient lighting
- energy efficient appliances
- dimmer switches
- power tools
- arcing on power lines
  - loose wires
  - tree branches touching
    power lines
- neighbors

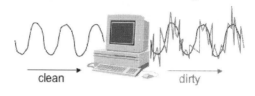
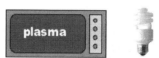

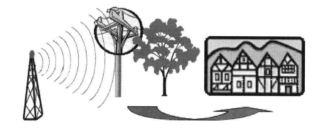

Dirty Power

#76. What is 'power quality'? And what is 'dirty power'?

MH: Power quality refers to the generation and distribution of electricity. In North America we generate a 60 Hz sine wave. The condition of the electricity is referred to as power quality. Dirty power is the noise that is imposed on the 60 Hz signal. The more the electricity deviates from the 60 Hz sine wave the poorer the power quality and the more 'dirty electricity'.

#77. Is the source of dirty power exclusively from RF emitting towers and RF emitting consumer products? Did the problem of dirty power exist prior to the cell phone industry?

MH: Any type of arcing or shorting caused by loose electrical wires or trees touching power lines will produce dirty electricity, so yes, dirty power existed prior to the cell phone industry. Dirty electricity became a serious problem in the 1970s as we began to use more electronic technology and went to energy efficient appliances and has continued to get worse because of aging infrastructure, growing use of wireless technology, etc. Some of the dirty power today, however, is a result of RF on the power lines.

#78. If I do not use a cell phone or any RF personal equipment, like a cell phone or portable phone, how serious is the impact on my electrical wiring from dirty power?

MH: If you have computers, plasma TVs, dimmer switches, fluorescent lights, energy efficient appliances and have neighbors who share your transformer, you will have dirty electricity in your home. Electricity comes into a home and goes through a final step down transformer that provides the proper voltage. Several homes are usually hooked up to the same transformer and they have similar power quality issues. A dimmer switch in one home can influence power quality in an adjacent home on the same transformer.

CR: A new peer-reviewed study worth reading on dirty electricity can be found at http://www.ncbi.nlm.nih.gov/pubmed/18512243.

It demonstrates a cancer cluster in a southern CA school with high frequency voltage transients and showed that RF in the kilohertz range carried on house and building wiring is a *potential universal carcinogen.* A single year of employment at this school increased a teachers' cancer risk by 21%, and if one were there more than 10 years the cancer risk increased by 610%.

Incandescent vs. Compact Fluorescent Light

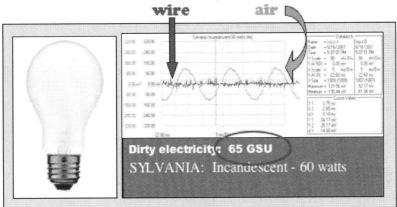

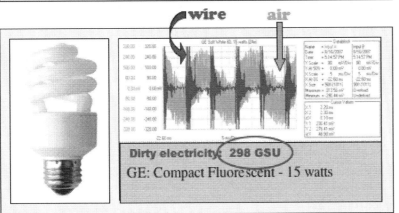

Compact Fluorescent Bulbs -

Hazards:

1. Mercury

2. Radio frequency radiation

3. Dirty electricity

4. Make people Sick

Science Re. 'Information Carrying Radio Waves'

#79. Can you explain more about why information carrying radio waves are different from regular waves? I want to defend this to my scientifically-minded friends who ridicule the idea.

MH: Dr. Ross Adey wrote that cells "whisper" to each other and their language is both chemical and electromagnetic. If these cells are then exposed to similar frequencies they may become confused and "get the wrong message" and hence react biochemically to the "false" information.

When we are transmitting many different frequencies, the probability there will be interference with cell function increases. This is a form of electromagnetic interference (EMI) that the industry is very concerned about when it interferes with radio stations, for example.

Satellites

#80. Does radiation from satellites pose similar dangers, or is it too weak?

MH: Satellites produce signals that are quite weak by the time they are picked up by "satellite dishes" or other receivers. Many people have a satellite dish on or near their home. The satellite dish at your home is a receiver and should have low levels of RF. The signals near these dishes are weak and should not pose a health threat. Some extremely sensitive individuals claim they can "feel" this radiation, however.

Underground Power Lines

#81. Are underground power lines as dangerous to our health?

MH: Underground wires do not have an electric field because it is blocked by the earth. They have a high magnetic field immediately above them but this decreases rapidly with distance. Generally underground wires is a good way to go but since it is expensive, the electrical utilities do not favor this option except for short stretches.

Ground Current

#82. I hear that the utilities are using the earth to return electrical currents to substations instead of returning the currents via neutral wiring. Are there health consequences?

MH: Another important source of electromagnetic pollution most lay people don't know about is called 'ground current'. In the early 1990s safety regulations governing the distribution of electricity were abandoned. Electrical currents that would normally go out over wires and return over wires now return to the substation via the earth underneath our towns, cities and rural areas. Electrical codes for safety were violated to avoid the costs of running more wire as demand expanded.

The result is that today we have farmers going out of business because their dairy cows produce less milk, miscarry or abort, have difficulty walking with swollen knee and ankle joints, and either waste away slowly or die suddenly.

People living on farms with a ground current problem have similar symptoms. Known health effects of ground current include cancers and miscarriages as well as chronic fatigue and chronic pain.

Ground current is not restricted to rural regions nor is it restricted to dairy farms. Dairy cattle, because they are milked at least twice daily, are equivalent to the 'canaries in the coal mine'. *They are telling us there is a serious problem and we better do something about it if we don't want to suffer the same consequences.*

In urban centers, our primary exposure to ground current is through plumbing. The more conductive the plumbing (metal vs. plastic) the more likely it will enter the home if it is present outside the home. Failure to provide sufficient capacity on the neutral wire combined with growing use of electronic devices and ageing distribution systems are the primary causes of this problem.

California is the only exception, where distribution of electricity via the earth remains illegal.

EMF exposure from ground current is another example of irresponsibility on the part of government who we expect are looking out for our health.

CR: For an eye-opening video showing the impact of ground current on dairy cows see, "*The Effects of Low Level Non-Linear Voltages and Frequencies Applied to Livestock"* available through Stetzer Electric (www.stetzerelectric.com). This video reveals how short cuts taken by utilities to avoid the expense of running more wire for the return of electricity causes very serious problems in animals, such as lowered milk production in cows, miscarriages, joint and foot problems, mastitis (inflammation of the udder in dairy cows), seizures and death, as well as sometimes very serious economic challenges for the farms. Human health problems are also a factor for people living on the farms affected.

Ground Current Problem on a Farm in Ontario, Canada

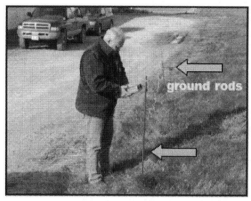

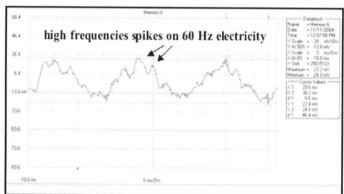

high frequencies spikes on 60 Hz electricity

- Low milk production
- Mastitis
- Foot problems
- Swollen joints
- Miscarriages
- Lower conception
- Odd behavior
- Tremors
- Sudden death

The above waveform was collected between two remote rods less than 20 feet apart on the Kerstendale farm near Port Perry Ont. The power to the farm was **off** at the time. (Dave Stetzer, 2004)

Big Picture

Responsibility for Current RF State of Affairs

#83. Who was responsible for getting Sec. 704 into the Telecommunications Act of 1996, which disallows state and local governments the right to influence the siting of towers on health/environmental grounds? Individual identities should be brought to light and people held accountable!

MH: Contact Janet Newton at www.emrpolicy.org

CR: Said to be the House Commerce Committee, as a last minute addendum written by lobbyists for industry. According to Janet Newton of the EMR Policy Institute Congressman Bliley in the House and Senator Pressler in the Senate worked out all the compromises in the bill. Here is the link to the Conference Report.

http://thomas.loc.gov/cgibin/ cpquery/?&dbname=cp104&sid=cp104TVz23&refer=&r_n=hr458.104&item=&sel=TOC_0 &

Attracting Media Coverage of this Issue

#84. I saw an article about cell phone use adding to commute time. Why are journalists not covering the serious health effects also? How can people help to make this FRONT PAGE news?

CR: Since the time of the Commonwealth Club event we are pleased to note major media is starting to cover this subject, including Larry King, the *New York Times* and others. If you know journalists who would benefit from receiving a E-copy of this document so they can get up to speed please let us know and we will send them a complimentary copy.

Also, see the *LA Times* story 3/25/08 by Myron Levin: "Cellphone Law May Not Make Roads Safer. Drivers Chatting, Even On Hands Free Devices, is Risky, Experts Say". This article discusses the subject of 'Cognitive Capture" that more journalists should be paying attention to, as well. Of note, in 45 countries today it is illegal to use a cell phone while driving (http://www.cellular-news.com/car_bans/).

Journalists need education before they will readily cover new topics. Consider sending an audio copy of the Commonwealth Club's EMF Panel 3/19 to journalists you know, or give them a link to the free podcast in the Commonwealth Club archive (www.commonwealthclub.org). As more journalists cover this emerging public health topic, more journalists will certainly jump in. But keep in mind that the newspapers, magazines and tv/radio stations that take advertising money from the wireless industry will have conflicts. Cases have occurred where a story on EMF/RF was in progress and management intervened to see it was not published.

The same financial conflict exists with our federal government, whose #2 source of revenue, it has been reported, comes from the telecom industry. These two conflicts of interest together (media and government) mean it is imperative that ***pressure come from the public for change***.

#85. You said youngsters using cell phones are at greatest risk—are you thinking about engaging the entertainment industry to reach kids? PSA on MTV of P. Diddy or Quincy Jones? Have you done outreach to engage popular icons?

CR: We would welcome creative ideas of how to get the message out to all constituents— children, parents, schools, the elderly, people with chronic illnesses, governments, etc. Forward your ideas of how you could help open creative doors to Camilla Rees at Camilla@ElectromagneticHealth.org. We would welcome collaboration with people in the entertainment industry who can make things happen fast.

#86. What efforts were made to the National Media so they could publicize the BioInitiative Report?

CR: So far, it seems the media coverage on the BioInitiative Report has not been strong, at least domestically. If you are in a position to help us fund a media campaign on the EMF/RF public health issue, including the science, and also the personal stories of how this issue is effecting peoples' lives, we'd be most grateful. We have many worthwhile communications projects looking for funding!

Philanthropists or foundations may contact Camilla Rees at Camilla@ElectromagneticHealth.org or call 415-992-5093. Request the document
"Funding Request for EMF/RF Awareness Raising, Education and Research."

Potential Consequences of Necessary Health-Protecting Changes for Industry and Consumers

#87. If the exposure standards are strengthened, what will be the effect on the communications technology industry? Will there be any reduction of services as a result?

MH: When the guidelines were discussed in Salzburg, the telecom industry said they could still function within these more limiting guidelines.

CR: Some people argue that if wireless services are not reduced, your health is simply not being protected. People need to learn what the science shows and only then, once they understand the gravity of what exactly is known about the health effects, decide what level of exposure is acceptable for society given the known risks. We must protect against the knee jerk response to want to protect our instant-gratification communications tools that we like very much ***at the expense of future generations.***

#88. How would we function—and compete—if we do away with wireless appliances?

CR: We have to acknowledge the truth of the health consequences within ourselves, and make decisions courageously to support life. From this place, we may also find solutions on the technological front. We will get nowhere, besides further illness, more damage to wildlife and increasing civil disobedience, if we continue to keep this issue under the rug.

The truth is, we lived very well before wireless technologies, and many would argue we lived much better, people seemed less fragmented, and more focused and present for work and relationships. Many people slept better, had less anxiety and depression, fewer neurological problems and heart diseases, less cancers, and so on. People who understand the importance of internal, human electromagnetic balance *believe we would be functioning much better if we were not bombarded by electromagnetic interferences from external sources!*

MH: We don't need to live without this technology, we just need to significantly minimize our usage of this technology. For example, you may need to use cell phones if you travel a lot but you do not NEED cell phones in your home. It is all a matter of degree.

That being said, we must at the same time be evaluating the long-term effects of these technologies, including the potential effects on future generations and the rest of the biosphere. We may discover alternative communications technologies are preferable from a human health perspective, and we must have the courage to adjust accordingly.

#89. Is fiber optic technology a viable alternative to Wi-Fi and are there any health consequences with fiber?

MH: Fiber optic is the ideal alternative. It has better security (others can't access the information as they can if it is wireless) and no radiation through the air. However, if wireless technology is used *within* the home there is still an issue. Fiber optics to the home/building and then *wired* routers provide the best alternative to wireless.

CR: Please note, some believe that possible health effects of fiber optic cables have not been fully explored, and while it does seems like the best option, we should make sure to do plenty of health impact testing before creating another multi-billion dollar industry and then finding out there is a problem. We need to insist on more thorough and comprehensive health testing of all technologies well before they are widely put into place.

#90. Is cable, combined with Wi-Fi into the home, safe?

MH: Using wireless increases radio frequency radiation. If there is cable present, why use Wi-Fi with it? Have the cable connection go direct into your computer or wired router.

CR: It takes relatively little effort to run the cable necessary to create a safe home environment, even if it means drilling small holes in the floor or ceiling, which can be concealed. Do not mindlessly accept the convenience of Wi-Fi at the expense of your health.

Also note that while Wi-Fi is more dangerous than cable; cable is not entirely radiation free. The FCC publishes emissions limits for coaxial cable, but these limits are designed for technology performance, not health, considerations. Cable companies are required to inspect cable for emissions regularly. There are amplifiers every few hundred feet along the cable and if these get loose there can be radiation leakage. You can check the cable in and around your house with a simple AM radio and see if radiation causes the radio to buzz. According to Stan Hartman, the stronger RF emissions will be very close to the cable, with some higher levels sometimes found around the input/output jacks of modems and routers.

#91. Has anyone looked at the psychological impact of wireless technologies in our lives?

CR: Chellis Glendinning, PhD, a psychotherapist and the author of six books, including *When Technology Wounds* and the forthcoming *Luddite.com: A Personal History of Technology*, says, "It never fails to amaze me the level of denial and psychic numbing—and gullibility—that surrounds what are in fact very dangerous, radiation-emitting technologies. Some people actually believe they can't live without them. Many have become dependent—truly addicted to them—and yet, let's face it, they have *only been using them for a few years.*" She adds, "The invasion by wireless technologies into the social-sphere has led not to personal connectivity and communication as advertised—but to alienation and isolation, less face-to-face community and cohesiveness, a speeding up of social relations, and a sense of 'placelessness'. On the collective level, this new electromagnetic infrastructure has led not to better democracy—but to increased centralization of political and economic power."

Glendinning adds, "According to our ancestors and a million years of evolution, mental health is rooted in knowing one's place and one's people. Historically, the foundation for well-being has been intimacy with family, tribe, culture, food production and the natural world. Today's mass society is already a world of individualism, displacement, factory food, and encasement in technology—and the new wireless technologies only further serve these predicaments; they hardly enhance family, tribe, local sustainability, or intimacy with nature. Look at the result! More mental illness, more thinking disorders, crime, depression, meaninglessness, violent behaviors like mass murders in public places, children killing children. Think about it."

#92. So, if cell phones are really this bad, what are the alternatives? Is it realistic to believe that all Americans would be willing to give up their cells, blackberries, i-phones, wireless, etc?

MH: It is all about knowing what your risk is and then deciding what you want to do about it. Some people are quite willing to take a risk if it has a benefit attached. Hence, even if someone thinks their cell phone has a chance of producing a brain tumor, they may take that "chance" and hope for the best. It is about information and choice.

CR: All Americans, of course, may not be ready and willing to give up these technologies. But it is more than an issue of individual choice, as these technologies are *blanketing society as a whole* whether one uses the technology or not. People are being subjected to involuntary radiation exposure, and lives are being harmed. We are impacting our collective health and the DNA and fertility of the species. Ethically, we must do the right thing.

Magda Havas, PhD remembers when x-rays were used to fit shoes, and radioactivity was used in ceramic pottery. Stan Hartman reminds us there was also a time when radium belts were used for backaches, and even radium toothpaste was the fad. There were also baby teething formulas with heroin, and Coca-Cola with cocaine. "What is it worth to prevent an epidemic of brain cancer, not to mention DNA changes that may affect all future generations?" he asks.

What is perhaps less realistic than the public giving up their addiction to these technologies is the U.S. government willingly putting the brakes on the wireless industry without a loud outcry from consumers. Not only is the telecom industry a major source of revenue for the U.S. government, but it has been reported that after the dot-com crash in the late 1990s, many companies who had purchased parts of the spectrum in the deregulation of the telecommunications industry did so with little money down, agreeing to pay the balance of the purchase price with user fees over time. As Dr. Joe Mercola's newsletter commented, "Essentially, the FCC is a mortgage holder for the mobile phone industry."

#93. What might be corporate interests in NOT setting protective limits?

CR: Throughout history, unintended consequences have frequently accompanied technological advances, such as with pharmaceutical, nuclear and coal mining technologies, for example, where there have been very serious human and environmental consequences, otherwise seen by society and scientists as 'advances'. Problems arise when there is a narrow focus on the technology, instead of appreciating the 'whole' impact. It is hard to put the brakes on once an industry is creating tremendous economic growth and jobs, and easier to put the blinders on, without very significant pressure from consumers or government. Of course, there are also potentially very serious liability issues, in this case, were industry to acknowledge previous limits on RF exposure were not adequate.

#94. Nearby Radar Station: There is an old navy radar station operating on Mt. Tam in Marin left from the Cold War era which scans the coast and operates 24/7. How much risk does it pose to health if you live in a home and can see Mt. Tam?

MH: Radar produces higher levels of microwave energy than cell phones and ideally your exposure should be measured to determine if you are at risk. Simply seeing it doesn't necessarily mean that you are exposed to unsafe levels.

CR: The radar beam may be scanning the coast, directed out to sea, or up in the air. There is no way to tell if the radar is a problem without directional measurements. The old navy radar is not the only thing on Mt. Tam of concern. The new Air Route Surveillance Radar (which looks like a golf ball the size of a house) is also of great concern and believed by residents to be causing ill health in several CA counties.

Exposure Standards Abroad

#95. Are the governmental standards in Europe and elsewhere more stringent than those in the U.S.? Are the acceptable levels for microwave, RF, etc in the US higher than in Europe?

MH: **Guidelines vary in orders of magnitude, with the UK having the worst guidelines and Salzburg, Austria having the best. The guidelines for the US are 4-fold worse than the ones in Salzburg.**

CR: See Section 3 of the BioInitiative Report (www.BioInitiative.org), The Existing Public Exposure Standards, including Chart 3.3, *Some International Exposure Standards of Cell Phone Frequencies (800-900Mhz)*, and also see Section 4, *Evidence for Inadequacy of the Standards*. As we went to print, Liechtenstein became the first country to commit to biologically based exposure standards in line with the BioInitiative Report, an exposure limit of 0.6 V/m.

#96. What precautionary steps have been taken abroad on this issue?

CR: There are signs of progress around the globe including: (1) the National Library of France deciding to dismantle wireless, in part based on the findings of the BioInitiative Report; (2) Germany advising against wireless in residential neighborhoods; (3) the dismantling of hundreds of towers in Taiwan; (4) stern warning from the Russian government on children's use of mobile phones and on use of mobile phones by pregnant women; (5) Israel restricting antennas on residential buildings, and cautioning that the specific microwave frequency at which cell phones broadcast utilize the human head as an antenna and the brain tissue as a radio receiver; (6) the European Environmental Agency advising use of the Precautionary Principle; (7) a Canadian university choosing to not have wireless; (8) schools in the UK removing wireless; (9) the International Association of Fire Fighters asking that antennas not be placed on fire halls until they are shown to be safe; (10) the chief of a 38,000 strong teachers union in the U.K calling for Wi-Fi in schools to be suspended due to reports linking it to loss of concentration, fatigue, reduced memory and headaches and the fear of its impact on children's developing nervous systems; (11) the European Parliament recently voting 522 to 16 that exposure guidelines need to be changed because they are 'obsolete'; (12) Liechtenstein announcing it will reduce exposure standards 10x to be within the BioInitiative Report recommendations, etc.

While there is more public and government awareness of the seriousness of this issue abroad than in the US, understand that precautionary steps taken abroad, while they look encouraging, mean very little in the face of the significant continued infrastructure build-out by the cell phone industry globally. *Major consumer pressure needs to be placed on governments worldwide to protect public health. And we need to recognize that, pending government action, that cell towers will not stop being built until people begin terminating their cell phone contracts in significant numbers.*

BioInitiative Report

#97. Where can we find a summary of the BioInitiative Report to provide to our City Council?

CR: www.BioInitiative.org. There is a summary for the public.

#98. Why are the results of the BioInitiative Report so different from the WHO's results? Isn't the output from a cell tower transmitter 50'-150' in the air comparable with output from over the air TV signals?

MH: There are two questions here. I'll answer the second one first: At the same distance from the antennas, the total output from a cell tower transmitter is much less powerful than from either radio or TV broadcasting or radar. It also uses different frequencies.

First Question: The two reports (WHO and BioInitiative) are based on similar studies but have different conclusions/interpretations. The Bioinitiative Report is based on the Precautionary Principle, which states that we err on the side of caution. It is asking for guidelines that are based on biological effects for extremely low frequency electromagnetic fields and for RFR, which are currently based on thermal effects only. In other words, if it doesn't heat the tissue it is considered safe by the WHO. This is a faulty assumption that has been discredited by scientific studies. Consequently the guideline needs to be changed to reflect the science and this is what the BioInitiative Report is requesting.

CR: Comparing cell tower and TV transmissions is comparing apples and oranges without knowing in each case how far away each is from the subject and what frequencies they are using.

Also, it is worth noting that WHO's ties to industry has previously been reported by Microwave News. http://www.microwavenews.com/nc_oct2005.html

#99. What has been the response of the EU and Germany?

CR: European countries have been much more concerned about this than the US. People are just beginning to appreciate the subject here. Officials in Germany, France, the UK and many other countries have issued warnings of different strengths, though no government has formally taken a stand until Liechtenstein in November 2008 mandated significantly lower emission standards by 2013. The National Library of France also recently announced they would dismantle the wireless in its libraries, exercising the Precautionary Principle, based in part on the findings of the BioInitiative Report. This was on the heels of the Paris library system dismantling wireless after 40% of the staff became ill.

In September 2008 the European Parliament voted 522 to 16 to reduce exposure to EMFs that have been linked to health risks. Noting the already lowered exposure limits in some EU countries, the European parliament is now calling on the EU council to amend Recommendation 1999/519/EC for all equipment producing emissions in the 0.1 MHz to 300 GHz frequency range. This would include cell phones as well as other wireless technologies.

In September 2008, The University of Pittsburgh Cancer Institute became the first medical center in the U.S. to take a precautionary stand on the hazards of cell phone radiation (http://environmentaloncology.org/node/201), followed shortly afterwards by Congressional hearings. We expect further attention to this issue in the U.S. as citizens learn more about the health effects and become activated around this issue.

Cell Phone Industry Response

#100. Do cell phone manufacturers or service providers acknowledge any health effects? Has anyone checked SEC 10k filings?

CR: Yes, telecommunications companies acknowledge potential health impacts in their 10k reports, the annual document required to be filed by public companies with the SEC. These documents are written by lawyers who know they have to tell the full truth, in contrast to annual reports which do not need to be as complete. You can find samples of recent 10ks of the telecom companies at www.emrpolicy.org or go directly to each company's own website. Names of telecom providers are conveniently listed at www.microwavenews.com. After reading the companies' 10ks, you will know there is *no uncertainty* about whether the cell phone companies understand there are serious alleged health consequences associated with their technologies and that the liability may be significant.

#101. What is the importance of the SAR value in assessing cell phone health risks? Why isn't this value available on the box so one can know it before purchasing?

MH: SAR stands for specific absorption rate and varies with source of exposure and subject using the phone. The exposure from your cell phone will depend on how close you are to an antenna and the absorption rate will depend on the person using the phone (size of head, distance from phone etc). Having said this, it is possible to standardize this metric and model the SAR for specific phones. If this was standardized and used by the industry it would provide at least some relative indication of exposure/absorption.

CR: Please note that the SAR value is not considered to be very helpful in determining the safety of a phone, as no one has ever measured the heat absorption rate inside an actual human head. It is also known that heat shock proteins appear in cells at exposure levels much lower than necessary to produce any heating (See BioInitiative Report- Section 7, Stress

Response). SAR values are created through simulation with head-shaped plexiglass filled with fluid, and many consider this assessment methodology to be inaccurate and irrelevant at determining the actual bioeffects of cell phones. SAR values of phones can be found at www.fcc.gov/oet/fccid using the FCC ID # on your phone or under the battery pack, but beware, as stated above, they are not of much value.

The Options Brief of the European Parliament's *"The Physiological and Environmental Effects of Non-Ionizing Radiation—Final Study"* states that "the efficacy of devices such as shields and ear pieces be indicated on the basis of biological tests, and not solely on the reduction of SAR value (as determined by use of a 'phantom' head) that their use might achieve."

While heating effects of a cell phone is considered insignificant compared to the radiation impact, it can indeed cause a temperature rise of up to 0.2 degrees Fahrenheit and there is a cumulative effect of the heating with prolonged or repeated use (*Health And Stress*, Newsletter of the American Institute of Stress, No. 6, 2008). There can also be hot spots created in the human head, even though on average the temperature rise may not be significant. If you are concerned about the heating effect, minimize use of your cell phone.

Why are Children More Vulnerable to Cell Phone Radiation?

Cell Phone Radiation Penetrating Skull

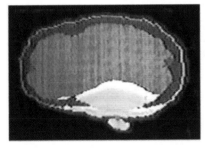 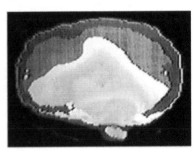

ADULT Head   **CHILD - 10 Years Old**   **CHILD - 5 Years Old**

Study by Gandi et al. University of Utah, 1996.

1. Children **absorb** more **energy** than adults from the same phone.

2. Tumors in **mid brain are** more deadly than those in **temporal lobe**.

3. Children's **cells** are **reproducing** more quickly than adults.

4. Children's **immune system** is not as well developed as adults.

5. Longer potential for **life-time exposure** for children than adults.

#102. How could the entire industry pretend there are only thermal effects—and get away with it for so long?

MH: Excellent question! The existing guideline is based on false assumptions that go unchallenged. We now have enough evidence to show non-thermal effects and need to convince those who set policy to re-examine this evidence and establish guidelines based on biological effects in addition to the thermal effects.

CR: Some people are comparing the current situation to what happened with tobacco—industry gets people hooked on the product so they won't want to hear about the dangers, then rake in the money until the dangers can't be ignored any more.

Advocacy for Change

#103. Is there an organized effort to amend the portion of the Telecom Act of 1996 that forbids consideration of health and environmental factors when placing towers?

CR: Please note that the Cellular Telephone and Internet Association (CTIA) has filed a petition to preempt local zoning authority over wireless sites, based on numerous undocumented claims about approval delays by local governments. The CTIA is essentially trying to strengthen the preemption clause of Sec. 704 of the Telecom Act of 1996. CTIA is requesting the FCC 1) force municipalities to act on wireless antenna or tower zoning applications within 45 or 75 days, 2) rule applications are deemed granted if a local government misses the deadline, 3) prevent municipalities from considering the existence of other carriers there in evaluating a carrier's application and 4) preempt any local ordinance that would require a variance for cell tower applications. If you are concerned about this further limitation of local zoning rights, we recommend people send comments to the FCC at Federal Communications, 445 12th Street, SW, Washington, DC 20554

ElectromagneticHealth.org has an **EMF Petition to Congress** specifically focused on returning state and governments rights, one of four points. Please sign it at www.ElectromagneticHealth.org!

To listen to a Congressional Staff Briefing on "Wireless and Broadcast Radiation Pollution" by the EMR Policy Institute, May 10, 2007, go to www.EMRPolicy.org where you may purchase this highly educational recording. To listen to testimony at the 1st Congressional Hearing on Cell Phone Use and Tumors September 25, 2008, visit http://domesticpolicy.oversight.house.gov/story.asp?ID=2199

Please note that Rep. Edward Markey, D-MA, is circulating draft legislation called the Wireless Consumer Protection and Community Broadband Empowerment Act. Its intentions are "To require the Federal Communications Commission to promulgate new consumer protection regulations for wireless service subscribers, to restrict state and local regulation of public providers of advanced communications capability and service, to increase spectrum efficiency by Federal agencies, and for other purposes." State laws governing the wireless industry would be preempted unless they were in line with federal laws. Overall, pro-consumer health groups see this as further reinforcing the federalization of telecommunications, and this draft legislation will need to be followed carefully. It will further compound the loss of our constitutional, civil and human rights that were taken away in Sec. 704 of the Federal Telecommunications Act of 1996 when government succumbed to industry pressure and facilitated the roll-out of radiation-emitting antennas nationwide before conducting an adequate, independent public health risk assessment.

None of this should come as a surprise when one looks at the size and strength of the telecommunications industry. The top 20 telecommunications companies have revenues approaching $1 trillion. Over the past decade it has been reported they have spent over $2.3 billion in political lobbying to influence government officials. We cannot rely on our government to protect the public health on this issue unless we bring the issue clearly in to light through public education. To support advocacy groups go to www. ElectromagneticHealth.org where, with one donation, you can support 6 leading non-profit groups working in this field in North America (EMR Policy Institute, International Commission on Electromagnetic Safety, Council on Wireless Technology Impacts, Citizens for Health Educational Foundation, National Institute for Science, Law and Public Policy and WEEP in Canada).

#104. What are the roles of the EPA, FDA, FCC and other federal government agencies with respect to protecting the public from the possible adverse effects of radiofrequency radiation? In other words, who is protecting us?

CR: With regards to the environmental effects of wireless transmitters, federal oversight is limited primarily to FCC regulation of radiofrequency signals coverage to ensure that licensed carriers can deliver clear signals and avoid mechanical signal interference among licensed carriers.

The FCC's radiofrequency radiation exposure standards governing exposure to radiofrequency radiation are protective against acute exposure and thermal heating effects from towers and antennas, but not against the effects of low-level intensity fields (those not likely to cause significant tissue heating), or against chronic/intermittent exposure, now routinely present in communities across the United States, or the constant exposure that will occur with Wi-Max.

The FCC guidelines were challenged in Federal court because, based on the science, these exposure standards are inadequate to protect health[1] but the U.S. Supreme Court did not accept the appeal.

No government agency is protecting us from acute or long-term, chronic exposure to the growing number of wireless transmitters, or from the known adverse health effects that

---

1   See Council on Wireless Technology Impact's press release and details on U.S. Court of Appeals challenge to the FCC's RFR human exposure guidelines and U.S. Supreme Court appeal at http://www.energy-fields.org/publicpolicy/litigation.html

are now showing up in the general population among early users of mobile telephony or among communities who live near antennas and towers or have installed them in their homes. In short, no one is assuring the traditional consumer protections we have taken for granted, nor granting citizens the right to know the possible adverse health effects of the electromagnetic field conditions to which we are being exposed.

In addition, the Telecommunications Act of 1996, Section 704, signed into law by President Clinton in February 1996, mandated that the Federal government will "prohibit state and local governments from restricting or influencing the siting of wireless antennas and towers based on environmental grounds.[2]" In fact, the telecommunications industry is entitled to sue cities and towns across America for failure to process permits to site antennas and towers on a timely basis or *if they are believed to have taken health into account when denying a permit application.*

This legislation essentially preempts our right to good health and affects the health of wildlife, domestic and farm animals and all living species, as well. A rapid wireless communication facility build-out has been effectively assured by fiat, and this situation will continue until that provision of law is repealed or declared unconstitutional. Absurdly, communities wanting to oppose antennas or towers on environmental grounds have to find technical reasons to justify denial, and are usually not successful. However through a process of grassroots education, more and more citizens are recognizing that their constitutional rights have been denied and are becoming more interested in challenging the laws that caused this to happen.

It will take an Act of Congress to redirect current practices by the Federal Communications Commission that has responsibility for licensing wireless transmitters. It is the citizen's job to bring Congress to enact remedial legislation. People wanting to put pressure on Congress to act to protect our health interests should sign the Petition "Urge Congress on EMF Safety" at www.ElectromagneticHealth.org.

Libby Kelley, Managing Secretariat of the International Commission for Electromagnetic Safety (www.icems.eu) and Founder of the Council on Wireless Technology Impacts (www.energyfields.org) advises, "It is important that people understand that the Federal government is not actively engaged in investigating potential or actual health risks related to electromagnetic field exposure from mobile telephones, laptop computers, Wi-Fi networks, Wi-Max and other wireless communications systems and personal devices. There has been a longstanding practice by the U.S. Congress and the Administration to provide limited resources to support the mission of Federal public health, worker safety, and environmental agencies to protect human health and safety and the natural environment. The result is, the current level of effort is not nearly equal to the task at hand and does not begin to address citizen and consumer requests for information and assistance."

---

2   See The Federal Telecommunications Act of 1996 (47 U.S.C. 332(c) (7) (B) (iv.)).

To empower an effective federal public health and environmental response, Kelley argues, "Congress must become much more motivated to take the health risks posed by wireless technologies more seriously than it is now". She says to do this would require that Congress act to:

1. **Authorize an independent, well-funded and sustained EMF research program** that coordinates federal public health agency research activities and provides continuing oversight and investigation;

2. Require the Federal public health agencies to **develop exposure standards that protect all biological systems;**

3. Require **exposure assessments and investigations** using a well-trained cadre of engineers and technicians who can do EMF testing upon request for the general public and for workers;

4. Require wireless and **electromagnetic product safety reviews and pre-market approval** by applying the Precautionary Principle until biologically based safety standards are in effect;

5. **Regulate disability access to public and commercial facilities and conduct routine inspections** to ensure cleaner indoor environments for persons who are functionally impaired due to electrical hypersensitivity;

6. Monitor and **investigate changes in wildlife biology and behavior** that may be caused or aggravated by electromagnetic field exposure;

7. Require frequent reports from the Administration; **hold public hearings to evaluate health effects, scientific and medical results**, and consider introducing remedial legislation.

When the Federal Telecommunications Act of 1996 was in development, according to Kelley, the Congressional Office of Technology Assessment was not engaged to perform a review of the potential impact on society. There also was no environmental assessment done by the Administration prior to enactment after a negative declaration determination was made under the National Environmental Policy Act. "Had this been done, many critical issues would have been raised," she says, "such as adverse effects of EMF on animals, trees and plants and the human health concerns that have been raised since by environmental groups. This includes evidence that EMF from wireless antennas and radio towers affect migratory bird behavior, and is resulting in a marked decline in certain species, and the growing number of people who report electrical hypersensitivity symptoms."

Kelley says that Federal agencies that historically have been delegated authority to perform such key programs and services have been curtailed by Congress, budget cutbacks, administrative orders or direct political interference. Examples cited include:

- The **U.S. Food and Drug Administration's** current position on cell phone safety dated July 29, 2003, is, "The available scientific evidence does not show that any health problems are associated with using wireless phones. There is no proof, however, that wireless phones are absolutely safe." The **U.S. Food and Drug Administration's Bureau of Radiological Devices** approved marketing of cellular phones in the early 1980s on behalf of U.S. consumers without first conducting a formal review of the available research on radiofrequency radiation, relying instead on the industry's view that there were no health risks without thermal heating of tissue. She says the FDA's research agenda has been heavily influenced and partially funded by the telecommunications industry. Given that 260 million Americans now are regular users of cell phone technology, it is imperative that the FDA act more aggressively to resolve these safety questions.

- The **U.S. Environmental Protection Agency**, which had the lead responsibility for research and investigation into civilian exposure to antennas and towers, saw its EMF research program terminated in 1985 and its exposure assessment and mitigation service closed in 1995, just prior to enactment of this major societal transformation initiated by new Federal telecommunications laws[3].

- The **National Institute on Environmental Health Sciences' National Toxicology Program**, according to Kelley, has been moving at 'glacial speed' in determining whether radiofrequency radiation is a human carcinogen or not, and, she says there are few Federally funded or direct Federal research programs underway in the U.S., independently of the industries that stand to benefit from a statement of "there is no credible evidence to demonstrate risk".

- The **National Institute of Environmental Health Sciences**, in conjunction with the **U.S. Department of Energy**, conducted a large extremely-low frequency EMF research program called EMF-Rapid in the mid to late 1990s, to evaluate scientific evidence that might link electrical and magnetic fields to adverse health effects. The study advisors reported a 'weak link' (meaning the evidence was merely based on epidemiological studies) between power line field exposure and childhood leukemia, yet Congress has still not held public hearings on these and other findings from that report[4].

3   Useful information about electromagnetic field safety provided by the U.S. EPA is at www.epa.gov/radiation/index.html. Click on 'Frequent Questions' in the column on the left. Then put in 'RF, EMF, cell phones' together as key words and press enter.

4   The EMF Rapid Report is no longer located on the NIEHS website but refers to http://www.niehs.nih.gov/health/topics/agents/emf/.

- The **FCC**, not a public health agency, acted to set uniform national radiofrequency radiation exposure guidelines for human health in consultation with industry-dominated standard-setting groups while ignoring significant comments made by key scientists in federal health agencies.

Kelley, an environmental and public health advocate who was a leading appellant in challenging the FCC's Radiofrequency Radiation Human Exposure Guidelines between 1997-2000, as well as co-producer of the documentary, *"Public Exposure: DNA, Democracy and the Wireless Revolution"*, says "The federal government's role in assuring the protection of human health or the natural environment when it comes to non-ionizing radiation exposure from cellular phones, other wireless devices, wireless transmitters, power lines or electrical equipment is non-existent and the existing exposure standards are irrelevant to real world exposure conditions. Chronic and involuntary exposure to non-ionizing radiation sources, including antennas, electrical wiring and from EMF emitting devices operating in and around schools, workplaces and homes are increasingly a part of our daily lives now."

Current concerns are over the Wi-Max roll-out, proceeding across the U.S without the slightest evidence of concern by our elected officials about its potential health impact, and Federal legislation in development that would place sole Federal regulatory authority for wireless transmitters under the FCC[5]. Plans for a national SMART electric grid with wireless communications components are also being widely supported for power quality and efficiency reasons, but are not considering health effects for the 3-8% of Americans already electrically sensitive, or the long-term impact on all others and on future generations. Broadband Over Power lines (BPL) will also bring another level of high frequency radiation exposure into each and every neighborhood, home, school and workplace, as will the move to energy efficient compact fluorescent light bulbs. It is clear—our government is asleep at the switch and not looking out for the impact of these new technologies on our health.

According to the newsletter of the American Institute of Stress, *Health and Stress*, published by Paul Rosch, MD, Clinical Professor of Medicine and Psychiatry at New York Medical Collage, "taxes on cell phone minutes are the government's largest source of consumer product revenue after gasoline" (www.stress.org). He also notes telecom securities represent a large percentage of the stock market, insinuating this sector will become vulnerable if government takes the kind of measures necessary to protect public health.

---

5   At the time of this report, Congressman Ed Markey is floating draft legislation, called "The Wireless Consumer Protection and Community Broadband Empowerment Act that would strengthen federalization of control over the wireless antenna and tower infrastructure and further compound the loss of our constitutional, civil and human rights, already preempted by Congress and the President when it enacted The Federal Telecommunications Act of 1996, as amended.

It is appropriate to question whether there is anyone in the Federal government looking out for our health! It appears the answer is 'No', as there is little to no official response to EMF public health problems reported to the FDA, FCC, EPA, the National Institutes of Health (NIH) and the Centers for Disease Control (CDC.)

In contrast, in May 2008, the EU adopted the position, by unanimous vote, that "the Precautionary Principle should be the cornerstone of the EU's policies on environmental health." According to Kelley, EMF risks were referred to as the chief example of risk. Mrs. Frederique Reis, a Belgian and member of the European Parliament stated, "*Where we delay in our reaction, prevention is the answer.*" In Fall 2008 the European Parliament voted 522 to 16 to update 'obsolete' exposure guidelines. The Venice Resolution, released in June 2008 by the International Commission for Electromagnetic Safety (www.icems. eu), urgently calls for more precaution until biologically based EMF exposure standards are in effect. That resolution is signed by peer reviewed, concerned scientists from all over the world.

While international awareness of serious health concerns is rapidly increasing, according to Kelley, the US government is said to be considering **relaxing the exposure standards in the U.S. even more.**

You are encouraged to contact your elected Federal and state representatives and express your personal health concerns, as well as concern about your right to know about the health hazards of man-made EMF exposure conditions in which we are increasingly being forced to live. Please take responsibility for ensuring that human health and life on our planet is preserved by signing the EMF Petition to Congress at www.ElectromagneticHealth.org.

New Technologies on the Horizon

#105. I hear long-distance Wi-Fi is coming soon, or 'Wi-Max'. It will blanket geographic areas for miles. What can we do if *we don't want this*? It seems to me this will put many sensitive people in jeopardy and contribute to the growth in the electrohypersensitive population. Who is looking out for our health?

MH: There is little any of us can do once Wi-Fi or Wi-Max antennas are installed. For those who do not want to be exposed to these frequencies it is essential they stop the antennas from going up in the first place. Unfortunately municipalities know little about the potential health effects of this technology and all they are aware of are the benefits for those who want to use their computers and connect to the internet. Wi-Max uses stronger antennas and is less desirable than Wi-Fi. Living near either type of antenna is undesirable, especially if you have developed sensitivity to these frequencies.

CR: People must start asking government where the *pre-market health testing* is for technologies using microwave radiation! Answers are long overdue. The multi-billion dollar Wi-Max collaboration (dubbed 'wi-fi on steroids') between Sprint, Clearwire, Time Warner Cable, Google and others will put the health of millions of electrically sensitive people in jeopardy.

I suggest you write Congress, your local government, local green building associations and start getting this in the minds of people locally. Without powerful and assertive action by health conscious individuals, the levels of radiation will dramatically increase across America by 2010, when half the antenna roll-out is expected to be complete. It has been reported Wi-Max antennas will cover 2 square miles, but further investigation shows they will have the strength to cover 38 square miles, to start. As one person said, "I am waxing nostalgic about how it used to be—when there was just concern about power lines and everyone was healthy and playing outdoors".

Folks, we are allowing our quality of life to be eroded by electromagnetic radiation by not questioning what is known of the health effects of these technologies. It will only get worse until we get involved. Please petition Congress to establish biologically-based exposure standards at www.ElectromagneticHealth.org.

A KPFA radio interview, *"WiMax: The Next Wireless Exposure"* (12/4/07) with Libby Kelley, Managing Secretariat of the International Commission for Electromagnetic Safety and Founder of the Council on Wireless Technology Impacts can be found at http://www.yourownhealthandfitness.org/ZenCart/index.php?main_page=product_info&cPath=68&products_id=1040 biologically-based exposure standards.

#106. What is 'Broadband Over Power' and is this something we should be concerned about? Does it mean radiofrequency radiation transmitted over the electrical wiring?

MH: Broadband over power lines (BPL) is a technology that enables transmission of broadband internet signals along ordinary power lines. Different frequencies in the radio frequency and microwave band of the spectrum are being tested and the ones selected will be those with minimal interference. In the future, BPL may be used with Wi-Max networks.

The unfortunate aspect of this technology is that it will bring these frequencies into the home on the electrical wiring. We already know that dirty electricity, frequencies other than 60 Hz, are making people sick. Studies of dirty electricity show an association with cancers, diabetes, multiple sclerosis, tinnitus, chronic pain, chronic fatigue, sleep disturbances, etc. Once broadband over power lines become operational a lot of people are going to become ill.

CR: People should be asking to see utility studies showing Broadband Over Power is safe. No one I know has seen any such studies, and given what is known about the health impact of radiofrequency radiation, the onus should be on industry to demonstrate safety before exposing populations to this technology. As we went to print, it was announced IBM has struck a deal with International Broadband Electric Communications to deploy BPL technology to electrical cooperatives that supply electricity to much of rural America.

L. Lloyd Morgan, BS, says "It is clear broadband over power will have major consequences because the electrical wires in our homes and buildings surround us on all sides—so it will be like being wrapped in a radio transmitter antenna". Lloyd is the author with Sam Milham, MD of the just released study on cancer connection with dirty electricity in a southern CA school, called "A New Electromagnetic Exposure Metric: High Frequency Voltage Transients Associated With Increased Cancer Incidence in Teachers in a California School", published in the American Journal of Industrial Medicine. The study found cancer strongly associated with high frequency voltage transients, which they concluded "may be a universal carcinogen, similar to ionizing radiation." (http://www.ncbi.nlm.nih.gov/pubmed/18512243)

According to one power industry expert, "The problem with BPL is that it will bring a signal into every home unless you install a filter at your incoming service, just like with internet on telephone services". As of yet, no such filters have been developed. Broadband Over Power is at higher frequencies than the 'dirty electricity' from RF on house wiring today, which as indicated above, has been linked to cancer. Graham Stetzer filters for dirty electricity only buffer frequencies between 4kHz-100kHz, and are not adequate for the higher frequencies of Broadband Over Power.

According to David Stetzer of Stetzer Electric, there is research dating back to the 1930s, also to be found in a book by utility industry expert witness, J. Patrick Reilly, showing any frequency above 1.7 kilohertz dissipates internal to the human body. Stetzer says there are 2 EPA report drafts on this still being held up by lobbyists, including "EPA. 1990. Evaluation of the Potential Carcinogenicity of Electromagnetic Fields. Review Draft: EPA/600/6-90/005B" and "EPA-SAB-RAC-92-013". Broadband Over Power would expose people to these damaging frequencies known to have health effects.

Sam Milham, MD, a medical epidemiologist in occupational epidemiology, confirms "There is a mountain of peer reviewed research showing that 'athermal' RF exposure is both biologically active and carcinogenic. Since the hazards are frequency dependent, the broadband signals are especially worrisome, compared to the power frequency fields. The broadband fields are alternating, man-made and of recent origin. There has been no time to evolve any defense." Dr. Milham was the first scientist to report increased leukemia and other cancers in electrical workers and to demonstrate that the childhood age peak in leukemia emerged in the U.S. in conjunction with the historical spread of electrification.

School Studies: Dirty Electricity & Cancer

Teachers' Cancer Cluster: La Quinta Middle School,
La Quinta, California (Milham and Morgan 2008).

Teaching in "hot" Rooms	Increased Cancer Risk
Never	80%
Ever	410%
Ever, >10 years at school	610%

#107. What are "smart meters" and do they pose a health threat. Can we opt out of using smart meters?

MH: A "Smart Meter" is the new way that the utility (both electric and water) wants to meter your use of this resource. Smart meters use radio frequencies to send information about your electricity use every few minutes back to headquarters. This enables variable pricing of electricity. The radio frequency may make some people ill, especially if they have developed sensitivity to these frequencies.

You can ask that the utility replace the Smart Meter with a regular mechanical hour-watt meter but you may have to pay the additional cost of having someone come out to manually read your meter. While this may reduce your exposure, other homes in your neighborhood will still be transmitting this information back to the utility every few minutes. This is yet another layer of EMR exposure that benefits the utility but not necessarily the customer.

CR: It is time for the green and sustainability movements to start considering the human health impacts of energy efficiency technologies, whether one is talking about utility meters and SmartGrids, Wi-Fi, Wi-Max or the health impacts of widely promoted compact fluorescent light bulbs, all of which emit radiofrequency radiation.

The best way to opt out is to become actively engaged with your government. Demand high standards for human health protection, and compassionate consideration for the growing number of people who have become electrically sensitivity. Please petition Congress at www.ElectromagneticHealth.org.

Also note, besides the health considerations of Broadband Over Power Lines, if combined with wireless there are also potential privacy and security issues, with strangers potentially being able to gain access to information about your patterns of utility usage.

Corporate Social Responsibility

#108. Has there been any outreach to educate corporations through the 'Corporate Social Responsibility' and 'Sustainability in Business' communities?

CR: Not that I am aware of. But this subject certainly should be brought to the attention of the more conscious business communities. Those who rank public companies on Corporate Social Responsibility measures should be encouraged to add Employee Electromagnetic Safety as a new evaluation criterion.

I recently visited a LEED certified new office building with the highest LEED certification. The building was beautifully designed, energy conscious, and the materials non-toxic, but the building had levels of EMF that were unsafe. Not only does the corporate world need to understand the effects of EMF on employee health and productivity, but so too, clearly, does the 'green building' movement.

In an interesting legal move, the EMR Policy Institute has filed formal opposition at the FCC to the Alltel/VWZ merger. Their Petition to Deny asserts the FCC has not addressed longterm exposure to radiofrequency radiation as required by the National Environmental Policy Act (NEPA). Worker safety, for 3rd party workers such as fire fighters, electricians, roofers, painters, window washers and other professionals who visit the wireless premises, is at issue. EMR Policy Institute's petition opposes the merger until a radiofrequency safety solution that protects all workers is implemented.

Legal Possibilities

#109. Halifax, VA became the 1st VA town to ban chemical and radioactive bodily trespass, stripping corporations of 'rights', announced 2/7/08. Community Environmental Legal Defense Fund Project Director, Ben Price, said "The people of the town of Halifax have determined that they do not consent to be irradiated, nor to be trespassed upon, by toxic substances that would be released by Virginia Uranium, Inc. or any other state chartered corporation. The people have asserted their right and their duty to protect their families, environment, and future generations. In enacting this law, the community has gone on record as rejecting Dillon's Rule, which erroneously asserts that there is no inherent right to local self government. The American Revolution was about nothing less than the fundamental right of the people to be the decision-makers on issues directly affecting the communities in which they live...The people of Town of Halifax have acted in the best tradition of liberty and freedom, and confronted injustice in the form of a state-permitted corporate assault against the consent of the sovereign people." Doesn't it seem that this approach is needed to protect us from the Telecom corporations?

JT: (Jim Turner, Esq., Chairman, Citizens for Health & Partner, Swankin-Turner in D.C.): This is an interesting phenomena. I have yet to see a corporate response to it. Generally speaking if Constitutional rights exist they cannot be eradicated by legislative action—any legislative action even by Congress. As a political move this is very exciting since if a significant number of communities across the country join this effort there would be a growing movement to cut back corporate power to effect individual lives. In my view, today we are in roughly the same situation with Large Multinational Corporations and the rights of individual human beings that we were in at the time of the American Revolution with regard to the relationship of the King and his government's relationship to individual human beings. To me, the antidote is to provide the same level (or more) of protection to the individual against corporations (which I consider at least quasi governments and in fact may be de jure governments since they have to have state permission to operate) that the Declaration of Independence, Constitution and Bill of Rights provide to human beings against governments. As legislation like the Halifax, VA ordinance move across the country, a movement to create protections of the individual against corporations picks up momentum. As I say, I have yet to see the corporate response to such a movement. Perhaps they are not yet taking it seriously.

#110. What can we as citizens do to restore state and local governments' rights to decide if we should be blanketed in wireless technologies? It seems like we don't have a chance anymore for health, and local governments, representing people, need to get involved.

MH: I suggest you contact your elected officials and get actively involved in the democratic process. Health-supporting changes will not occur until 1) the federal government changes microwave radiation exposure standards, with pressure from citizens, and 2) state and local governments' rights to influence the tower and antenna approval process is returned.

CR: To write to Congress, go to www.congressmerge.com/onlineb/index.htm or sign Electromagnetic Health's Petition to Congress at www.ElectromagneticHealth.org. We highly encourage you to take action. Also, please ask your doctor to report cases of electrohypersensitivity to the Department of Health so they can better understand the scope of this emerging health problem. And to whatever degree you are able, please support the worthy non-profits working in this field. With one donation at www.ElectromagneticHealth. org, you can support the efforts of 6 non-profits—The EMR Policy Institute, Council on Wireless Technology Impacts, International Commission for Electromagnetic Safety, National Institute for Science, Law and Public Policy (NISLAPP), WEEP Initiative in Canada and Citizens for Health Education Foundation.

How many people in this room have experienced adverse health effects from wireless emissions?

Estimated 70-80% by show of hands.

"Our lives begin to end the day we become silent about things that matter."

— Martin Luther King, Jr.

V. Books, Videos, Journals & Websites, etc.

Books

Cell Towers: Wireless Convenience or Environmental Hazard edited by B. Blake Levitt, Safe Goods/New Century Publishing, 2000

Electromagnetic Fields: A Consumer's Guide To The Issues And How To Protect Ourselves, B. Blake Levitt, Harcourt Brace, NY, 1995.

Silencing the Fields, Ed Leeper

The Body Electric: Electromagnetism and the Foundation of Life, Gary Selden, Robert O. Becker, Maria D. Guarnaschelli (Editors), William Morrow & Company, NY, 1987.

Cross Currents: The Perils of Electropollution, the Promise of Electromedicine, Robert O. Becker, M.D., Tarcher/Putman, NY 1990.

Warning: The Electricity Around You May Be Hazardous to Your Health, Ellen Sugarman

The Invisible Disease: The Dangers of Environmental Illnesses Caused by Electromagnetic Fields and Chemical Emissions, Gunni Nordstrom

Zapping of America: Microwaves, Their Deadly Risk and Cover-Up, Paul Brodeur

Currents of Death: Power lines, Computer Terminals and the Attempt to Cover Up Their Threat to Your Health, Paul Brodeur

The Microwave Debate, Nicholas H. Steneck

EMF Handbook, Steven Prata

Tracing EMFs in Building Wiring, Karl Riley

Health & Light, John Ott

Bioelectromagnetic Medicine, Paul Rosch (Ed.) and Marko S. Markov (Ed.)

Biological Effects of Electric and Magnetic Fields, DO Carpenter and S Ayrapetyan, Eds., Academic Press, San Diego, CA
Vol. 1 Sources and Mechanisms
Vol. 2 Clinical Applications and Therapeutic Effects

Bees, Birds and Humans-The Destruction of Nature by Electrosmog (booklet), Ulrich Warnke (in German only at present by the name "Bienen, Völker und Menschen"), 2008 bienenbroschuere@kompetenzinitiative.de

Silent Fields, The Growing Cancer Cluster Story When Electricity Kills, Donna Fisher (www.silentfields.com)

Web Sites

ElectromagneticHealth.org – www.ElectromagneticHealth.org

EMR Policy Institute, VT – www.EMRPolicy.org

Microwave News website – http://www.microwavenews.com/

Collaborative for Health & the Environment, EMF Working Group – http://www.healthandenvironment.org/

EMF Facts Consultancy Website – http://www.emfacts.com/

Council on Wireless Technology Impacts – http://www.energyfields.org/

EMR Network – http://www.emrnetwork.org/

WEEP/The Canadian Initiative to Stop Wireless, Electric and Electromagnetic Pollution – http://www.weepinitiative.org/

International Commission for Electromagnetic Safety – http://www.icems.eu/
(See Venice Resolution announcement 6/10/08 - *"Scientists Urgently Call for Greater Precaution to Protect Health from Pervasive EMF Exposure Hazards until Biologically Based Standards are In Effect".)*
http://www.icems.eu/docs/Venice_Resolution_press0608.pdf,

EM-Radiation Research Trust (UK) – http://www.radiationresearch.org/

The Swedish Association for the ElectroSensitive – http://www.feb.se/index_int.htm

Powerwatch (UK) – http://www.powerwatch.org.uk/

Mast Action (UK) – http://www.mastaction.co.uk/

H.E.S.E. Project (UK) – http://www.hese-project.org/heseuk/en/main/index.php

Antenna Search Database (find where antennas are in your neighborhood) – http://www.antennasearch.com/

WiFi in Schools – http://wifiinschools.org.uk/

Videos

Electromagnetic Radiation: A Scientific Overview, by Dr. Theodore Litovitz, physicist, Catholic University of America. (VHS/PAL 25 min.) Watch on www.ElectromagneticHealth.org.

Public Exposure: DNA, Democracy and the Wireless Revolution - First place award at the Santa Cruz Earth Vision Film Festival, 2001 and in 2008 won best documentary. (VHS/PAL 58 min.) Watch on www.ElectromagneticHealth.org.

CBS News - YouTube Video on Cell Tower Disguises — http://www.youtube.com/watch?v=uRQYan_-CTQ

ABC Good Morning America Video on Electrohypersensitivity — http://abcnews.go.com/Video/playerIndex?id=3289424

BBC News Video on Health Risks of Wi-Fi in Schools — http://news.bbc.co.uk/player/nol/newsid_6680000/newsid_6680400/6680481.stm?bw=nb&mp=rm&news=1&ms3=0&ms_javascript=true&bbcws=2

Congressional Staff Briefing on "Wireless and Broadcast Radiation Pollution" by the EMR Policy Institute, May 10, 2007, www.EMRPolicy.org

Congressional Hearings on Cell Phones and Tumors, September 25, 2008 http://domesticpolicy.oversight.house.gov/story.asp?ID=2199

The Effects of Low Level Non-Linear Voltages and Frequencies Applied to Livestock www.stetzerelectric.com

Journals

Electromagnetic Biology and Medicine

Bioelectromagnetics (Bioelectromagnetics Society — www.bioelectromagnetics.org)

Journal of Pathophysiology — special issue on EMF, 3/09

Measuring Devices & Other Resources

EMFSafetyStore.com — http://www.EMFSafetyStore.com

Alpha Lab Inc. — http://users.maui.net/~emf/

Safe Living Technologies Inc. — www.safelivingtechnologies.ca

Technology Alternatives Corp. — http://www.drgauss.com/

"Facts don't cease to exist just because they are ignored."

— Aldous Huxley

"Liberty can not be preserved without general knowledge among people."

—John Adams

Section VI – Community Health Survey

The Green Audit
Community Health Assessment

The following page contains a questionnaire called the **Green Audit**. It is important when administering the **Green Audit** that you work with someone trained in epidemiology, and also not disclose to respondents that the questionnaire will be measuring anything related to the technologies in question. Please send copies of your data collected, when complete, to the EMR Policy Institute, PO Box 117, Marshfield, VT 05658.

We recommend you consider conducting a 'before and after' Green Audit community health survey:

1) If a **new cell phone tower** goes up in your neighborhood,

2) If your utility company implements **Broadband Over Power** technology carrying RF fields onto the electrical wiring in buildings, or

3) In anticipation of 'involuntary' **24/7 Wi-Max radiation** in your community, reported to be rolling out across America and to cover half of our country by 2010. Wi-Max is a joint venture including Sprint (NYSE: S), Clearwire (NYSE: CLWR), Intel Capital (NASDAQ: INTC), Time Warner Cable (NYSE: TWC), Brighthouse Networks, Google (NASDAQ: GOOG) and Comcast (Nasdaq: CMCSA, CMCSK).

Conduct the survey initially, and then 3-6 months after the event.

THE GREEN AUDIT: Health Questionnaire

Code: ____ | office use only

Please complete this questionnaire and return it to: | P.O. Box 117, Marshfield, VT, 05658 | by: ____

INSTRUCTIONS: This health questionnaire has 10 questions. You will be invited to complete this questionnaire twice: once now and again within the next few months. The purpose of the questionnaire is to determine any changes in your health status during this period. While the results will be published, your identity will remain confidential. We ask you to identify yourself (with initials) only so we can compare your first and second questionnaire responses. If you are a business location, please feel free to copy the questionnaire for all employees willing to participate.

---

1 Gender: male ☐ female ☐   **2** Birth: month ☐ year ☐

3 Check as many as apply: I sleep ☐ work ☐ at the location this questionnaire was delivered.

4 Document the frequency and severity of any of the following during the past month.

	frequency			severity			Symptoms are . . . than normal.		
	rare	sometimes	often	mild	moderate	severe	better	same	worse
headache	☐	☐	☐	☐	☐	☐	☐	☐	☐
poor short-term memory	☐	☐	☐	☐	☐	☐	☐	☐	☐
tremors	☐	☐	☐	☐	☐	☐	☐	☐	☐
dizziness	☐	☐	☐	☐	☐	☐	☐	☐	☐
depression	☐	☐	☐	☐	☐	☐	☐	☐	☐
blurred vision	☐	☐	☐	☐	☐	☐	☐	☐	☐
difficulty sleeping	☐	☐	☐	☐	☐	☐	☐	☐	☐
irritability	☐	☐	☐	☐	☐	☐	☐	☐	☐
difficulty concentrating	☐	☐	☐	☐	☐	☐	☐	☐	☐
fatigue	☐	☐	☐	☐	☐	☐	☐	☐	☐
chronic pain	☐	☐	☐	☐	☐	☐	☐	☐	☐

5 Do you currently have any of the following medical conditions and have symptoms changed during the past month?

6 During the past month symptoms are . . . than normal.

	no	yes	if "yes" →	better	same	worse
Amyotrophic Lateral Sclerosis	☐	☐		☐	☐	☐
Alzheimer's Disease	☐	☐	if "yes" indicate type	☐	☐	☐
Cancer	☐	☐	type: ____	☐	☐	☐
Diabetes	☐	☐	type: ____	☐	☐	☐
Heart Ailment	☐	☐	type: ____	☐	☐	☐
High Blood Pressure	☐	☐	→	☐	☐	☐
Multiple sclerosis	☐	☐	type: ____	☐	☐	☐
Parkinson's Disease	☐	☐		☐	☐	☐
Immune System Disorders	☐	☐	→	☐	☐	☐
Other? Please specify	____			☐	☐	☐

7 Check which of these electronic devices you use in your home and/or at work and the frequency of use.

	at home			at work		
	never	sometimes	often	never	sometimes	often
cellular phone	☐	☐	☐	☐	☐	☐
cordless phone	☐	☐	☐	☐	☐	☐
wireless computer network	☐	☐	☐	☐	☐	☐
baby monitor	☐	☐	☐ type	☐	☐	☐ type
other wireless devices (speakers, etc.)	☐	☐	☐	☐	☐	☐

8 Please provide your initials (or pseudo initials) in the box to the right so that your answers to the first and second questionnaire can be compared. ☐

9 Today's Date: ☐

10 (Optional): Additional comments about your health can be provided on the back of this questionnaire.

Section VII - Links to Petitions—Endorse ElectromagneticHealth.org's Petition to Congress, The BioInitiative Report and The Venice Resolution

1) EMF Petition Congress to:

> **1)** Change exposure standards so they are biologically based,
>
> **2)** Return state and local governments' rights to limit wireless antennas on health and environmental grounds,
>
> **3)** Declare a moratorium on further wireless infrastructure build-out, including Wi-Max, and
>
> **4)** Establish wireless-free zones and wireless free schools.

Please sign at www.ElectromagneticHealth.org

2) Endorse the BioInitiative Report, which recommends biologically-based exposure standards. Please sign the petition of the EMR Policy Institute at: http://www.ipetitions.com/petition/bioinitiativeemrpi/

3) Scientists and Physicians Please Endorse The Venice Resolution, at www.icems.eu. See Press Release 6/10/08: *"Scientists Urgently Calling for Greater Precaution to Protect Health from Pervasive EMF Exposure Hazards until Biologically Based Standards are in Effect".*

It is only through the government hearing from you about this emerging public health issue that progress to protect public health can be made. Please sign the petitions ASAP.

"Never doubt that a small group of thoughtful, committed people can change the world. Indeed, it is the only thing that ever has."

— Margaret Mead

"All truth passes through three stages. First, it is ridiculed. Second, it is violently opposed. Third, it is accepted as being self-evident."

— Arthur Schopenhauer

Section VIII - How to Support Further EMF Advocacy & Research

If you are able to support this important public health issue, please let us know.

Funding is Needed Now For:

- **Educational Efforts**
- **Government Advocacy**
- **Creating & Implementing Solutions**
- **Scientific Research**
- **1st Conference of Scientists, Physicians & Philanthropists**

Educational Efforts

- ***Health practitioners need to be trained*** *to identify electromagnetic factors in health so they can properly diagnose and then help their patients.*

- ***Communities need well trained remediation experts*** *to assess and remediate home and office environments.*

- ***Consumers*** *themselves, especially those with chronic illnesses, need education so they can take an active role in creating healthy environments.*

- ***Schools and libraries*** *need to be educated on the effects of microwave radiation on attention, behavior and learning.*

- ***Parents need to understand*** *the concerns about long-term radiofrequency exposure for children.*

- ***Health practitioners need to be educated on EMF-drug interaction,*** *such as diminishing efficacy in breast cancer therapies, as well as EMF interference with critical care therapies, such as pacemakers.*

- ***Fertility experts and patients trying to conceive*** *need to learn of the negative impact of electromagnetic factors on fertility, as well as in miscarriage.*

- ***Nursing homes, retirement living centers and seniors*** *need education on the importance of this issue to their cognitive function and physical health.*

- ***Known wildlife and atmospheric impacts need to be shared with environmental organizations*** *so they, too, can respond to this issue as their own.*

- ***Government and corporate health executives*** *need to appreciate the significant EMF/RF connection with health costs.*

Government Advocacy

- **Exposure standards** *need to be corrected at the federal level so that they are biologically based.*

- **The FCC Act of 1996, Section 704,** *which rescinded state and local governments' rights to influence the siting of towers and antennas on "environmental" (including health) grounds, needs to be repealed so that local decision making authority about tower and antenna permits is restored to local communities.*

- **Communities and/or governments need to review present antenna health hazards,** *beginning with residential neighborhoods and schools.*

- **Communities need to be educated that wireless networks are especially inappropriate for residential areas,** *and then follow the lead of countries that have banned or advised against installation of wireless in residential areas.*

- **Wireless technologies should be banned in public learning environments,** *such as libraries and schools, following the lead of the National Library of France.*

- **Americans With Disabilities Act protection** *is needed for patients who are functionally impaired.*

- **Legal counsel committed to this issue is needed to support local activists** *across the country fighting wireless in public buildings, citywide Wi-Fi and tower placements, as well as to initiate a class action suit against the FCC by people whose lives have been harmed.*

- **Governments and industry need to stop promoting Compact Fluorescent Bulbs** *as a 'healthy/green' alternative to incandescent bulbs, since high frequency RF radiation emitted by CFLs cause very significant negative health impacts for millions of people. Energy efficient LED bulbs that cause none of the health consequences, and are even more energy efficient than CFLs, should instead be the bulb of choice, with research funds allocated to their further development.*

- **"2nd Hand Radiation" protection** is needed so people who are electrically sensitive can have full access to society, including schools, libraries, residential neighborhoods, stores, transportation, hospitals, conferences, courthouses, and all other government buildings, without becoming ill.

Creating & Implementing Solutions

- **Plans to complete the extensive national fiber optic infrastructure, without the health effects of Wi-Fi, needs to be put on the front burner,** *and other technology alternatives encouraged.*

- **Communities need safe places of refuge for those most severely impaired,** *including comprehensive health recovery oriented services.*

- **A diagnostic category** *for radiowave sickness, or electrosensitivity, should be established, embracing present reality fully, so that this impairment receives recognition as well as funding to better help those who are suffering.*

- *Corporations concerned about productivity and employee health* need to clean up their high 'electrosmog' environments impacting employees.

- *Full disclosure to tenants should be required* where wireless transmission equipment has been installed on, in or in close proximity to apartment buildings.

- *Full disclosure of the presence of nearby antennas in residential real estate sales* should be required, including antenna locations and wattage.

- *Expansion of Green Building and LEED standards* to include EMF/RF considerations.

- *Moratorium on any further antenna sitings, including the Wi-Max roll out,* until the government's evaluation of long-term, chronic exposure to wireless devices is completed.

- *Legal support for churches, schools and others wanting to break contracts* with industry where hazardous antennas have been sited on their property.

Scientific Research

- *Public and private research funding* as recommended by the BioInitiative Report, International Commission for Electromagnetic Safety and other independent scientists.

- *Compile the evidence for ELF/RF connection with different diseases* so it is readily accessible by the media, government and others.

- *Research on human DNA impact; brain damage; all neurological conditions; and to establish the clear connection with chronic illnesses driving health costs.*

- *Follow up on initial studies that showed increased mortality, and increased morbidity, after antenna systems are built in a neighborhood.*

- *Research into the RF connection with bee colony collapse, mold growth, the obesity and diabetes epidemics, and chemical sensitivity.*

Strategic Communications Team

- *A core team of leading scientists, physicians, advocacy groups, philanthropists and communications professionals must gather and strategize to accelerate change in a coordinated way,* by activating the public, politicians, government officials, foundations, businesses, health practitioners, and environmental and other allied organizations. This is a critical issue that needs coordinated action now.

- *If you can help to financially support activists in this field,* please contact Camilla Rees at Camilla@ElectromagneticHealth.org or (641) 715-3900 Ext. 61768#.

Thank you!

Bios/Photos of Authors

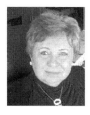

Magda Havas, PhD. Dr. Havas is Associate Professor of Environmental & Resource Studies at Trent University, Canada, where she teaches and does research on the biological effects of environmental contaminants, including radiofrequency radiation, electromagnetic fields, dirty electricity and ground current. She has served as expert witness on matters dealing with electrical pollution in both Canada and the United States, and has been advisor to non-profits, including Wireless Electrical and Electromagnetic Pollution in Canada, Council on Wireless Technology Impacts and EMR Policy Institute in the U.S., HESE in the U.K. and National Platform Stralingscrisco's in the Netherlands. Dr. Havas recently prepared a 50-page scientific analysis on the potential adverse health and environmental impacts of a proposed citywide Wi-Fi initiative in San Francisco. Her report recommended an environmental review be conducted, and the application of the Precautionary Principle, before rolling out city wide wireless in San Francisco.

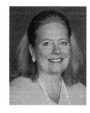

Camilla Rees, MBA. Ms. Rees is CEO of Wide Angle Health, LLC, a patient education and advocacy organization. She combines 15 years of business experience in investment banking, venture capital and marketing communications with 12 years as an active student and teacher of health optimization. She is presently writing her next book, on health care reform, and developing marketing strategy for health care, environmental, natural products and social change organizations.

The questions answered in this document were raised by attendees at the Commonwealth Club's panel, **"Microwave Radiation: The Shadow Side of the Wireless Revolution"** on March 19, 2008. The full panel included **Magda Havas, PhD, Cindy Sage, MA, David Carpenter, MD, MPH and Camilla Rees, MBA.**

This public affairs event was sponsored by the Commonwealth Club of California's Environment & Natural Resources and Health & Medicine Member-Led Forums, and co-organized by Wide Angle Health, LLC in association with Citizens for Health, a leading consumer health advocacy organization and the American Academy of Environmental Medicine.

No endorsement of the contents of this document by the above organizations and individuals is implied. Answers to questions posed by attendees at the Commonwealth Club panel are solely those of the individual authors, as indicated, and reflect our best understanding of the science at this time.

To listen to the audio recording of the Commonwealth Club presentation go to www.ElectromagneticHealth.org

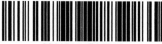

Made in the USA
San Bernardino, CA
10 September 2016